T0383571

ROUTLEDGE LIBRARY EDITIONS: SLEEP AND DREAMS

Volume 7

SLEEP AND AGEING

SLEEP AND AGEING

KEVIN MORGAN

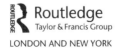

Routledge
Taylor & Francis Group

LONDON AND NEW YORK

First published in 1987 by Croom Helm

This edition first published in 2018
by Routledge
2 Park Square, Milton Park, Abingdon, Oxon OX14 4RN

and by Routledge
711 Third Avenue, New York, NY 10017

Routledge is an imprint of the Taylor & Francis Group, an informa business

British Library Cataloguing in Publication Data
A catalogue record for this book is available from the British Library

ISBN: 978-1-138-23090-3 (Set)
ISBN: 978-1-315-10370-9 (Set) (ebk)
ISBN: 978-1-138-23291-4 (Volume 7) (hbk)
ISBN: 978-1-315-31101-2 (Volume 7) (ebk)

Publisher's Note
The publisher has gone to great lengths to ensure the quality of this reprint but points out that some imperfections in the original copies may be apparent.

Disclaimer
The publisher has made every effort to trace copyright holders and would welcome correspondence from those they have been unable to trace.

SLEEP AND AGEING

Sleeping patterns change with age, whether we are growing up, or growing old. While most people are prepared for the rapidly altering sleep patterns of growing children, the evidence suggests that many are unprepared for additional sleep changes in later life, either in themselves or in others. In this book two research disciplines — social gerontology and sleep research — are brought together with the aim of providing a straightforward account of how sleep is changed and disrupted by the biological and social impact of ageing. Attention then focuses on the personal and clinical response to these changes. The use of sleeping drugs among elderly people is critically examined, and effective alternatives, including self-help practices and psychological therapies, are described. The influence of ageing on the recall and content of dreams is also considered. In the final chapter, the author comments on current styles of responding to sleep problems in old age and discusses the need and the scope for change.

This book deals with topics of universal interest and provides valuable information for those professionally as well as personally concerned with sleep quality in later life, including health professionals (nurses, doctors, psychologists etc.) working with elderly people, gerontologists, and sleep researchers.

SLEEP AND AGEING

KEVIN MORGAN, PhD,
Department of Health Care of the Elderly,
University of Nottingham Medical School

CROOM HELM
London & Sydney

© 1987 Kevin Morgan
Croom Helm Ltd, Provident House, Burrell Row,
Beckenham, Kent BR3 1AT

Croom Helm Australia, 44–50 Waterloo Road,
North Ryde, 2113, New South Wales

British Library Cataloguing in Publication Data

Morgan, Kevin
   Sleep and ageing: a research-based guide
   to sleep in later life.
   1. Sleep   2. Aged
   I. Title
   612'.821'0880565   RA786
   ISBN 0–7099–3578–1

To Sarah and Luke

Typeset by Photoprint, Torquay, Devon
Printed and bound in Great Britain
by Billing & Sons Limited, Worcester.

Contents

Acknowledgements

In preparing the manuscript for this book I have been helped directly by the advice and guidance of specific individuals, and also indirectly by the experience gained as a research worker in two quite different academic environments. First, then, I would like to thank those colleagues past and present in the Department of Psychiatry, University of Edinburgh, and in the Department of Health Care of the Elderly, University of Nottingham, who have helped to stimulate and foster many of the ideas presented here.

Much of the research I have undertaken, particularly that described in Chapters 4 and 5, has involved teamwork, and I am pleased to acknowledge the contribution and support of my collaborators who are named in the text. Thanks are also due to Dr David Harrod for commenting on the manuscript and, as ever, for helping me with the English language, to George Seaton for his expert help with the word processing software, and to Dr Chris Gilleard for constructive and enjoyable discussions on the topics covered in this book, and for his advice and comments on their presentation. Finally, special thanks are due to Maureen Tomeny for her encouragement, support and constructive criticism throughout the preparation of the manuscript.

Introduction

In the first few months of life healthy human infants spend about 17 hours out of 24 fast asleep. The sleep of these babies is not concentrated into one period of time, but is distributed throughout the day and night with episodes of sometimes quite noisy wakefulness intervening. By the time the process of maturation is complete the now adult human spends, on average, about seven and a half hours asleep each day. All of this sleep is concentrated into one period of time (usually at night), and sleep at any other time is considered unusual and socially undesirable. By the seventh and eighth decades of life many healthy individuals will sleep for less than six hours each night, few will experience the continuous unbroken sleep of their earlier adult years and, for some, daytime napping will become both habitual and satisfying. Patterns of sleep change with age, whether we are growing up or growing old. Nevertheless, while most people appear to be prepared for the rapidly altering sleep patterns of growing children, the evidence suggests that many are unprepared for additional sleep changes in later life, either in themselves or in others.

In this book two research disciplines, sleep research and social gerontology, are brought together with the aim of providing a straightforward account of how sleep is influenced by the biological and social impact of ageing. In doing so I have made certain assumptions which are reflected in the content and organisation of the first three chapters. I have, for example, assumed that the terms of reference of academic sleep research will be less familiar to the reader than those of gerontology — the study of human ageing. Accordingly, Chapter 1 is concerned with describing the historical development and explaining the current use of techniques for measuring aspects of sleep and wakefulness. Throughout the text I have also tried to keep the day-to-day jargon of research to a minimum, and where necessary terms are defined or clarified as they are used.

Having identified factors which contribute to age-related changes in sleep, later chapters focus upon and examine the personal consequences of these changes. Sleep disturbance in later life is inextricably linked with the issue of sleeping drug usage. Chapter 4 provides much of the background to this assertion, and after briefly describing what sleeping drugs are and what they do, goes on to examine critically the extent to which these drugs are used among elderly people. Disadvantages associated with the use of sleeping drugs among elderly people are described in Chapter 5, while Chapter 6 considers some alternative strategies for coping with problem sleep in old age. It should be noted that this book is not intended as a do-it-yourself therapeutic manual, however. For many people the topics of sleep and dreams are also inextricably linked and in Chapter 7 two aspects of dreaming in old age — the recall of dreams and the content of dreams — are given brief consideration. In the final chapter, I offer a critique of some of the issues raised, and suggest ways in which current styles of responding to insomnia in old age might change.

For the most part (with the exception of the final chapter) I have tried not to stray too far from straight and narrow conclusions drawn from research findings, though it is sometimes difficult to avoid occasional conjecture. While the material considered here was selected from an extensive and ever growing literature, I have attempted to include the most important or the most representative studies, or to emphasise the most relevant controversies. It has not, however, been my intention to produce a definitive academic text. My overall goal has been to provide an informative and readable book of value to those professionally or personally concerned with sleep in later life.

1

The Study of Sleep

Towards the end of a career that spanned almost 60 years, Ivan Petrovich Pavlov, eminent Russian physiologist, member of the Royal Society and Nobel prize-winner, concluded that sleep was a relatively straightforward process characterised by 'spreading cortical inhibition'. By this Pavlov meant that as brain cells fatigue, they switch off one by one. When enough of them have switched off the brain falls asleep.[1] Conversely, as each cell becomes restored, then it switches back on and, when enough are switched on, the brain awakes. For Pavlov there was no single structure in the brain which controlled these events; the states of sleep and wakefulness were democratically selected by the cells of the cortex. While many scientists in the early decades of this century may not have agreed with the detail of this view, most shared the assumption that sleep was a fairly simple process during which individuals passed into a state of unresponsive somnolence, where they steadily remained until full consciousness returned. As all good scientists ought to be at some point in their career, Pavlov was wrong. It is now widely accepted that sleep is not only a complex, but also an active process. Far from 'switching off', activity in the cortex (that part of the human brain responsible for so-called higher activities like thinking and solving problems) sometimes becomes quite intense even though the individual is sleeping soundly. Characteristics of sleep unrecognised by experienced scientists in the early 1920s have now become common scientific knowledge.

This improved understanding owes much to two developments which ultimately revolutionised the study of sleep. The first of these concerned the way in which sleep was quantified or measured, while the second concerned the way in which these measurements were subsequently interpreted. The significance of these two developments are probably best understood in a historical context.

THE MEASUREMENT OF SLEEP

Traditionally, interest in sleep has been related to interest in dreams. It is unsurprising, therefore, that in the late nineteenth century interest in the nature of sleep received an indirect stimulus from the psychoanalytical movement which, under Freud, held dreams to be the rational organisation of unconscious thoughts, interpretable through analysis, and deserving of much attention. Psychoanalysts not only brought their attention to the study of dreams, they also brought their method — science. By the early years of the twentieth century what might be identified as sleep research consisted of the disparate but occasionally overlapping interests of physiologists, psychologists, psychiatrists, and others. Sleep is not a single event but at least to the researcher is myriad coordinated events and processes, any one of which may be measured and analysed. Aspects of the sleeping state selected for measurement reflected more or less the background of the researcher. Thus, while physiologists measured variations in blood pressure, temperature, heart rate and blood chemistry etc., those with a psychological bent showed a preference for the behavioural nature of sleep, for example its depth, its duration, or the effects of sleep loss on the mental state.

By the early 1930s considerable information had been accumulated concerning biological events during sleep, the periodicity or time schedule of sleep, and also the physiological and psychological consequences of sleep deprivation. Despite the large amount of information produced it was clear to some researchers that something was missing. Simply put, between sleep as described by the scientists, and sleep as experienced by the individual, there existed a credibility gap. At the level of human experience, sleep is not assessed in terms of fluctuations in temperature, or changes in systolic blood pressure. Rather, we tend to consider sleep in terms of its duration, its depth, its restorative quality and so on. What was conspicuously absent from sleep research at this time was an adequate means for relating the objectively measured processes of sleeping to the personal experience of sleep. What was required was a measurement, or a cluster of measurements which reflected relevant physiological change, and also correlated with sleeping behaviour.

To this end, considerable attention had focused upon movement, and elaborate electro-mechanical devices had been developed for quantifying (with considerable accuracy) the frequency and duration of gross body movements during sleep. All night records of motility, or 'actogrammes',[2] could be compared with an individual's report of sleep quality, or could be used to contrast the sleep of one individual with that of another. Because movement in bed is frequently related to our experience of 'restful' or 'restless' sleep, actogrammes could also be used to assess, in a meaningful way, the effects of sedative drugs on sleep. This would provide a clear link between the physiological effects of a drug (in terms of reduced motility) and the psychological consequences of taking the drug (in terms of more 'restful' sleep). While useful, the actogramme had many limitations, not least of which was its inability to record the moment at which sleep began or when it ended, neither of these events being accompanied by characteristic patterns of movement. Indeed, at this time there existed no adequate means at all for detecting when sleep onset or when waking actually occurred. Consequently, not even the most popularly used characteristic of sleep, its duration, could be determined with complete accuracy in the laboratory.

Electrical brain activity and sleep

The first of the two developments which radically changed this state of affairs had, at the time, little to do with sleep research. In 1925 Hans Berger, Professor of Neurology and Psychiatry at the University of Jena in central (now East) Germany, recorded electrical brain waves from wires attached to the scalp of his young son. [Such recordings are made by a pen or stylus resting on a moving and markable surface. Amplified electrical discharges cause oscillations of the pen resulting in a trace similar in kind to those shown in Figure 1.1. In the figure the pen has moved up and down while the paper has moved from right to left.] While it had long been recognised that nerve

3

Figure 1.1: Electroencephalogram (EEG) tracings of sleep stages recorded from a young adult

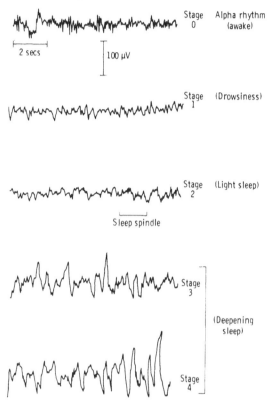

tissue produces tiny electrical discharges when at work, these discharges had only previously been recorded from the exposed brains of animals. Professor Berger, however, was concerned to find the physiological origins of psychic phenomena in general, and telepathy in particular and, possibly for this reason, showed more interest in the activity of human brains.[3] Coupled with this discovery was the further observation that the frequency and amplitude of the recorded waves could be influenced by loud noises, closing the eyes, or by concentrating, each of these events producing distinctive and recognisable wave forms. In the first report of this work published in 1929, Berger chose the term 'Elektrenkephalogramm' to describe his recordings. The term persists today, and the English form – electroencephalo-

gram – is frequently reduced to the more manageable 'EEG'.
Berger's results were not immediately accepted by the
scientific community. This (not untypical) scepticism gradually
gave way as interest in the Austrian psychiatrist's recordings
grew, and further research replicated his original findings.
Nevertheless, it took several years before the relevance of the
EEG to the study of sleep was recognised. In 1935 Alfred L.
Loomis and colleagues working in New York reported that the
electroencephalogram of the sleeping human shows four quite
distinct patterns which they named 'random', 'saw-tooth',
'trains', and 'spindles', depending on the appearance of the
wave.[4] By comparing these EEG patterns with simultaneously
measured breathing rate, pulse and motility, these researchers
rather cautiously concluded that 'a change in the level of
consciousness was connected with this change in type of wave.'
For example 'trains' were associated with settling down and
falling asleep, while the slower 'random' activity appeared to
predominate when sleep was deeper. This rather tentative
conclusion, that EEG, behavioural and physiological events are
synchronised during sleep provided the basis for much subsequent (and most contemporary) sleep research, and marked the
beginning of the second major development which greatly
influenced the study of sleep, the interpretation of the sleeping
EEG.

Brain waves and the structure of sleep

The EEG appeared to provide a method capable of measuring
the onset, progress, and depth of sleep. Further research by
Loomis and his colleagues[5] identified a total of five wave forms
typical of normal human sleep which, on the whole, seemed to
correlate with the sleeping individual's level of consciousness.
These wave forms, variants of the originally identified 'random',
'saw-tooth', 'trains', and 'spindles', they labelled A, B, C, D
and E 'in order of appearance [during sleep] and in order of
resistance to change by disturbance [from lightest to deepest]'.
It was also apparent from the EEG records that an individual
did not simply descend to 'deep' sleep and stay there until
awakened (as, for example, Pavlov had assumed), but rather,
after progressing through each state of sleep from A to E,
lighter sleep would return rather abruptly and the sequence

would start again in cyclical fashion. In other words, levels of consciousness or awareness appeared to fall and rise again several times during the course of normal sleep.

The assumption persisted for several years that changes in the characteristics of the EEG represented qualitatively different levels of consciousness in the sleeping human with low voltage fast activity typifying light sleep, high voltage slow oscillations typifying deep sleep. Nevertheless, it was apparent to some researchers that this relationship did not always hold, and that some low voltage activity could accompany profoundly deep sleep. Prominent among the scientists who utilised the electro-encephalograph for detailed studies of sleep was Dr Nathaniel Kleitman working in the Department of Physiology at the University of Chicago. In 1953 Eugene Aserinsky, a research student at the Chicago laboratory, together with Kleitman, published a brief report in the journal *Science*[6] which not only provided a more appropriate interpretation of the all-night EEG, but also stimulated immense interest in the enterprise of sleep research.

Concerned mainly with eye-movements during sleep, Aserinsky and Kleitman had extended their EEG apparatus to include an electro-oculogram (EOG), which recorded electrical activity from plate electrodes placed above, below, and on either side of both eyes. These electrodes, very similar to those used on the scalp, are sensitive to changes in electrical potential between the cornea and the retina such as occur when the eye moves. Thus, the electro-oculogram provided a continuous record of eye movements throughout sleep. From the resulting EEG and EOG recordings, these researchers reported that, at regular intervals throughout the night, the usual slow rolling eye movements associated with sleep (and clearly visible beneath the closed lid) gave way to bursts of rapid conjugate eye movements lasting from one to several minutes. Synchronous with these bursts of rapid eye movements were low voltage, irregular brain waves — the EEG pattern characteristic of light sleep — and an increase in pulse and breathing rate. Rapid eye movement episodes occurred sometimes three, and occasionally four times each night and lasted for, on average, 20 minutes. The average interval observed between these episodes was about one and a half to two hours, this interval getting shorter as the night progressed. The feature of Aserinsky and Kleitman's report that aroused most interest, however, was the finding that, if woken during a rapid eye movement period, individuals would more likely than not report dreaming. If woken during sleep without the rapid eye movements, individuals were unlikely to report dreaming. The observable onset and duration of rapid eye movement sleep indicated the onset and duration of the sleeper's dream experiences.

Once again, interest in dreams stimulated interest in sleep. By the early 1960s the findings of Aserinsky and Kleitman had been replicated on numerous occasions in laboratories throughout the world. Among the conclusions drawn from these many studies was that the EEG activity associated with Rapid Eye Movement (or REM) sleep represented not just a quantitatively different level of consciousness (i.e. 'deeper' or 'lighter' sleep), but a qualitatively different *type* of sleep. Following upon the work of Kleitman and his colleagues in Chicago one further characteristic of the REM state has been described which completes the now commonly used electro-physiological profile of sleep. In 1961 Ralph Berger, a sleep researcher working in the Department of Psychological Medicine at the University of Edinburgh, reported that during REM sleep the muscles of the neck show a profound degree of relaxation.[7] From appropriately placed electrodes similar to those used for EEG and EOG measurements Berger had hoped to monitor any attempted speech in his sleeping subjects by recording the electrical activity in muscles (electromyograms or EMGs) over the larynx. In fact, the EMG showed a marked reduction in muscle activity consistent with relaxation immediately prior to the occurrence of rapid eye movements which was then followed on the EEG trace by the characteristic low voltage irregular brain waves. Further research showed that this relaxation associated with the REM period was also present in the trunk and limbs, and the additional measurement of muscle (usually chin muscle) activity, in combination with the electroencephalogram and the electro-oculogram, further refined the ability of researchers to distinguish between REM and non-REM sleep and has since become standard in most all-night recordings.

The Polysomnogram

In 1968 internationally agreed criteria for interpreting the 'polysomnogram' (i.e. the EEG, EOG, and EMG recordings made during sleep) were published.[8] These criteria, incorporating the accumulated wisdom of 40 years of brain-wave recording, remain in use today, and describe five 'stages' of sleep. The four stages of non-REM (or NREM) sleep are identified principally on the basis of EEG appearance, and are very similar to those reported by Alfred Loomis and his colleagues in 1935, while the fifth stage, REM, is usually identified on the basis of combined EEG, EOG, and EMG activity. The EEG patterns typical of these stages are shown in Figure 1.1. Incidentally, since first being described by Aserinsky and Kleitman, REM and NREM sleep have attracted numerous epithets. REM sleep has not uncommonly been referred to as 'paradoxical sleep' (because the EEG suggests light sleep while the individual is, in fact, quite deeply asleep), 'dreaming sleep', or 'active sleep'. NREM sleep, on the other hand, has been termed 'orthodox sleep' or 'quiet sleep'. Whatever the descriptive merits of these terms, REM and NREM will be used preferentially here.

When the subject is relaxed (but with the eyes closed) the EEG is characterised by alpha waves, mixed voltage activity with a frequency of 8–13 cycles per second. Stage 1 sleep, drowsiness, is accompanied by lower voltage mixed frequency activity which may appear haphazard or 'desynchronised' or may be regular and 'synchronised' at about 4–6 cycles per second. The onset of light sleep is determined by the appearance of stage 2, mixed voltage activity of the alpha type showing clear episodes of 12–14 cycles per second 'sleep spindles'. Stages 3 and 4 accompany 'deep sleep', and are frequently subsumed within the single term 'slow wave sleep' or SWS. These slow waves are of high voltage, with a frequency of between 1–4 cycles per second, the slower and more uniformly high voltage pattern being characteristic of stage 4. The EEG of REM sleep is, as already explained, similar to that of stage 1. However, unlike any other sleep stage it is also accompanied by episodic rapid eye movements and profound relaxation of the muscles which maintain posture (the so-called anti-gravity muscles of the limbs and trunk) both being events clearly visible on the EOG and EMG traces. REM sleep is also accompanied by phases of quite intense physiological activity: the pulse rate quickens, blood pressure rises, respiration rates increase, and oxygen consumption is higher than at any other time during sleep. In adult males REM sleep is further associated with the occurrence of penile erections, a sometimes uncomfortable event which, as will become clear in Chapter 2, is not without its implications for sleep continuity.

A typical laboratory analysis of sleep involves the continuous recording of EEG, EOG, and EMG from the onset of sleep to final awakening. The resulting record, which may be ink traces on paper or digital information on magnetic tape, is interpreted or 'scored' using the criteria outlined above. The order and duration of each sleep stage is calculated, and the frequency of shifts from one stage to another computed. A convenient way of graphically representing the structure of a single sleep period is shown in Figure 1.2. The time spent in each stage is represented by horizontal lines, while the vertical lines indicate a shift from one stage to another. (In reality, these shifts are a little less abrupt than the diagram suggests). As was suggested by the earliest EEG recordings, and confirmed by subsequent studies, sleep stages follow each other in a cyclical fashion. Having progressed through the NREM stages 1 to 4, an individual may then return, stepwise, to stage 2 before the first REM period begins, after which the same cycle starts again.

The all-night polysomnogram provided researchers with a tool capable of quantifying many aspects of sleep which earlier had proved so elusive. The moment of sleep onset, the total duration of sleep, the number and duration of any awakenings during the night, and a great deal more can be determined from a single recording. Measurements of sleep which are commonly derived from the all-night electroencephalogram are summarised in Table 1.1.

Measuring depth of sleep

Much more so than the measurement of physiological change or bodily movement, the EEG also provides some insight into the *quality* of sleep likely to be reported. The number of stage shifts, for example, (see Figure 1.2) indicate to some extent the degree of restlessness during sleep. A typically restless night would involve many such changes from one sleep stage to another. With this type of measurement the gap between sleep as described by the researcher, and sleep as experienced by the individual is greatly reduced. Other methods of quantifying aspects of sleep, used in conjunction with EEG measures, have reduced the gap even further. Some of these methods have

9

Table 1.1: Measurements of sleep derived from the all-night electroenecephalogram (EEG)

Sleep Onset Latency. The time taken from the decision to go to sleep (or, in the laboratory, from 'lights out') to the appearance of the first stage of actual sleep (stage 2).

Sleep Period Time. The time from sleep onset (q.v.) to final awakening.

Wakefulness After Sleep Onset or Intervening Wakefulness. Episodes of (usually 30 seconds or more) stage 0 that occur within the sleep period. Intervening wakefulness can be expressed in terms of *duration* (e.g. total minutes of wakefulness) or *frequency* (e.g. number of awakenings per night). In either case, wakefulness of this type indicates the degree of sleep disturbance.

Frequency of Stage Shifts. Transitions from one sleep stage to another are referred to as stage shifts, and are frequently associated with gross body movements. The number of shifts observed during the sleep period can also be used as a measure of sleep disturbance.

Total Sleep Time. This refers to the period from sleep onset to final awakening (i.e. the sleep period) minus any intervening wakefulness. Because periods of significant wakefulness are deducted, total sleep time is a rather pure measure of the actual duration of sleep.

Duration of Each Sleep Stage. The time spent in each sleep stage during a single night can be expressed either in units of time (e.g. total minutes of stage 1, etc.) or as a percentage, usually of the sleep period time (this allows for the calculation of the percentage of intervening wakefulness).

Time in Bed. While fairly meaningless in laboratory situations where the times of going to and getting out of bed are frequently imposed, the time spent in bed becomes particularly important when individuals are permitted to 'free run' and select their own time of arising. Time in bed is usually defined as the period from 'lights out' (i.e. settling down to sleep) to rising.

Sleep Efficiency. The proportion of time in bed actually spent asleep is frequently used an an indication of sleep *efficiency*. Defined as total sleep time divided by time in bed, this measurement assumes that if someone is in bed, then they are at least trying to get to sleep.

---

particular relevance for an understanding of age-related changes in sleep, and therefore deserve special mention.

Most appreciate the metaphor of 'deep' sleep, it refers to sleep from which the individual is not easily aroused. While methods for measuring depth of sleep have been recognised for over a century, the meaningful interpretation of these measurements had to wait until the 'EEG era' had begun. In 1860 Gustav Theodor Fechner, erstwhile professor of physics at the

Figure 1.2: Diagrammatic representation ('Hypnogram') of sleep stages (typical pattern for a young adult)

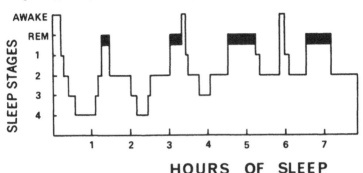

HOURS OF SLEEP

Note: Horizontal lines represent the time spent in each sleep stage, while the vertical lines indicate 'shifts' from one stage to another. In this way the cyclical nature of sleep is clearly shown. Darkened areas represent REM periods.
Source: Kales *et al.*, UCLA Interdepartmental Conference on Sleep and Dreams, *Annals of Internal Medicine*, Vol. 68 (1968) pp. 1078–1104. Reprinted with permission.

University of Leipzig, described in his text 'Elemente der Psychophysik'[9] a method for assessing depth of sleep by measuring the minimum intensity of a stimulus necessary to wake a sleeping individual. Variations in the required stimulus intensity corresponded to variations in depth of sleep. The minimum intensity of a given stimulus required to wake someone is referred to as its awakening or arousal threshold value; if the chosen stimulus is some form of noise (for example a tone or a bell), then this threshold is called the auditory awakening threshold and may be measured in decibels. Early attempts to measure auditory awakening thresholds during sleep produced disappointingly inconclusive results. Arousal thresholds appeared not only to differ greatly between individuals, but also appeared to vary enormously within the same individual. As these fluctuations could not be accounted for, the measurement of awakening thresholds during sleep was not pursued with much enthusiasm, and for many years was totally ignored. With the introduction of EEG measures, however, the source of these fluctuations soon became apparent. As implied by Loomis and colleagues in 1935, each identifiable stage of sleep is associated with a different awakening threshold. The

11

intensity of an auditory tone required to wake a sleeping experimental subject, for example, is greatest in stage 4, slightly less in stage 3, and least in stage 2. REM sleep presents a rather special case but, in terms of the auditory awakening threshold, is at least as 'deep' as stage 4. Thus, arousal thresholds which were once dismissed as unreliable measures are now regarded as one the most meaningful ways of quantifying depth of sleep.

Measuring subjective characteristics of sleep

As already suggested, the description of sleep now provided by the EEG and collateral measures relates quite easily to our own experience. Ways in which we commonly regard our own sleep, including its depth, duration, and the time it took us to 'drop off' are all accurately (in fact, much more accurately) assessed by the EEG. One aspect of our sleep to which no instrument has direct access, however, is our personal appraisal of its quality. Sleep possesses both subjective and objective character-istics. While the EEG describes the objective 'observable' characteristics of the sleeping state in a practical and meaningful way, it cannot quantify the experience of sleep quality. We may refer to 'good' sleep, or to a 'good night's sleep' but we don't necessarily mean a long sleep, or a continuously unbroken sleep, or even a rapidly achieved sleep. Sleep with which we feel satisfied on awakening is good sleep, and sleep with which we feel dissatisfied on awakening is not good sleep. Because of the personal introspective nature of these judgements, the only realistic way of assessing the quality of someone's sleep is to ask them about it. The easiest way of doing this, of course, is simply to inquire of the individual concerned whether they are satisfied or dissatisfied with the quality of their sleep. Variations on this question have been used to great effect in the population surveys to be considered in later chapters. No matter how systematically asked, such questions are a little bit like rulers which have only two graduations, big and small; they are better than nothing at all, but are also of limited usefulness.

More sophisticated measures of sleep quality have been developed in response not so much to the needs of research into sleep as such, but to the needs of research into the effects of certain drugs upon sleep. For reasons possibly more related to the sociology of medicine than the physiology of sleep, the use of sleeping tablets increased steadily throughout the post-war period and, by the mid 1960s sleeping drugs were among the most popularly prescribed of all medicines.[10] The bulk of these prescriptions were for hypnotic (sleeping) drugs of the barbiturate type which, while clinically very effective, possessed at least two highly undesirable characteristics. Barbiturates had an unacceptably high abuse potential, and were unacceptably toxic in overdose. To this, the pharmaceutical companies responded by developing 'non-barbiturate' hypnotic products (some of which were even less desirable than the drugs they aimed to replace). Aware of the need to demonstrate the effectiveness of these new products relative to the well-tried and (at least as sleep inducers) reliable barbiturates, the drug industry turned to sleep researchers for a thorough evaluation of the hypnotic properties of new sleeping drugs. Sleep laboratory 'trials' of hypnotic drugs became, and remain, the definitive test of a putative sleeping drug's efficacy. Evaluating the effects of sleeping drugs not only provided sleep research with a wealthy patron in the form of the pharmaceutical industry, it also provided a stimulus for broadening the measurement of the subjective characteristics of sleep.

Essential for a product which has to find favour with prescriber and public alike, a successful hypnotic drug must not only induce and maintain sleep effectively, it must also allow for the recipient to awake feeling *satisfied* with that sleep. No matter how effective at the objective level, few will want to continue taking a drug which, at the subjective level, makes them feel dreadful the following day. Simple questions which achieve only a 'bigger–smaller' type of measurement do not permit detailed comparisons between, say, two drugs both of which may improve sleep quality, but one relatively more than the other. Nor does the simple question detect gradual improvements, or decrements, in sleep quality over many nights. Clearly, the more precise measurement of subjective states related to sleep required a more sophisticated approach to questioning. Multiple-item questionnaires which, when completed, yield a numerical score provide one answer. Sleep questionnaire scores from different individuals, or from the same individual on different occasions, can be used to compare the subjective quality of sleep during one night with that during another. Check-lists of adjectives relating to feelings and mood have also been used, the subjects 'checking' (i.e. ticking) the words which they think describe appropriately their mood or feelings at the time the list is completed. Lists may be constructed such that higher scores indicate satisfaction with sleep and feelings of early morning tranquillity, while low scores indicate dissatisfaction with sleep and feelings of irritability. Again, each list, which may be presented on many occasions, provides the researcher with a numerical score.

Perhaps the most elegant device that has been used for assessing the subjective characteristics of sleep is the simple visual analogue scale.[11] This usually consists of a ten centimetre straight horizontal line with opposing statements at either end (e.g. 'my best night's sleep ever' on the left and 'my worst night's sleep ever' on the right). The subject of the assessment is asked to place a mark on the line at a position which, in their opinion, corresponds to their feelings about the previous night's sleep. A mark in the centre represents a fairly average night, while a subsequent tendency to mark to the right would indicate a subjective decline in sleep quality, and a drift to the left would indicate improvement. Thus the visual distance between these marks is analogous to the perceived 'distance' between subjective feelings on one morning, and subjective feelings on another — hence visual analogue scales. Each separate mark can be given a numerical score by measuring the distance in millimetres from, say, the left side of the line to that day's mark. When completed daily over a period of weeks or months, these simple and easily understood measurement scales provide a sensitive record of any changes in the subjectively experienced characteristics of sleep.

Night-time sleep and daytime behaviour

The measurements considered so far focus almost exclusively on events which occur during, or immediately following, a single night of sleep. It must be remembered, however, that sleep itself is not isolated from our waking lives. Evolution has synchronised biological and solar events such that, in the absence of environmental or physiological disturbance, the alternating states of sleeping and wakefulness are accommodated within, and controlled by, an approximate 24 hour rhythm, the circadian rhythm. Sleep both influences, and is influenced by, the behaviour of this fundamental biological timekeeper. If the rhythm is disturbed as, for example, in jet-lag or shift work, then sleep is disturbed. Conversely, if sleep is inadequate, then waking performance will be characterised by tiredness and inefficiency. Despite the intimacy of the inter-relationship between sleeping and waking, measurements of the latter have been relatively neglected until recent years. Growing interest in the nature and consequences of poor sleep, together with a need for increased rigour in assessing the effects of sleeping tablets, prompted researchers at Stanford University in California to develop a method for objectively measuring *sleepiness*. It is interesting to note that over the years a tradition had evolved among sleep researchers who, when describing or simply referring to the state of sleepiness, elaborately avoided the use of subjective, colloquial and (supposedly) 'unscientific' language. It was not unknown to find scientists virtually apologising for using such terms as 'fatigue', preferring instead such phrases as 'conditions which develop under circumstances of prolonged arousal'.[12] The principle guiding the choice of terminology here is, in fact, fairly simple — to define a concept scientifically, refer only to what is observable. Put more formally, the definition should be stated in terms of the procedures or operations involved in establishing or measuring the defined concept. This type of definition, called an 'operational definition', actually originated in physics and was subsequently adopted by scientific psychology in the 1930s and 1940s. It is precisely because 'sleepiness' can be defined operationally that it has come, at least in sleep research, to replace 'fatigue', 'drowsiness', and 'tiredness' etc. as the description of choice for that state which results from loss of sleep. Sleepiness refers to a tendency to fall asleep. The test developed at Stanford, the Multiple Sleep Latency Test (MSLT),[13] assesses this tendency by measuring the time taken for an individual connected to an EEG machine to fall asleep (the Sleep Latency) while lying on a comfortable bed in a quiet darkened room. The sleep latency can be defined in various ways, for example the time that elapses from 'lights out' to the first occurrence of 30 continuous seconds of stage 2 sleep, or to the first 90 seconds of stage 1. Whatever definitional criteria are used, interpretation of the measure remains the same, the longer the sleep latency, the less sleepy the subject. This procedure may be repeated throughout the day and night, if necessary providing a contiguous account of daytime sleepiness. So as not to disturb subsequent measurements, individuals are, of course, woken shortly after achieving their quota of criterion sleep.

SLEEP RESEARCH AND THE ELDERLY

Assessed in terms of the number of experiments reported in scientific journals, interest in sleep research and in the application of EEG-related measurement techniques expanded rapidly following the discovery of REM sleep. One aspect of sleep which attracted a lot of attention was ontogenetic change, that is, normal change throughout the course of life from infancy to old age. As knowledge accumulated, research was able to document in a systematic way what had been realised probably for hundreds of years, that the sleep of the elderly is markedly different from the sleep of the young. Nevertheless, for many years the sleep of older individuals was a very low research priority. Having recognised that the sleep of the young and the old were frequently quite different, many sleep researchers reflecting traditional social values, tended to regard the sleep of younger adults as 'normal', and virtually excluded older individuals from sleep experiments. Until quite recently, for example, laboratory studies evaluating the effects of sleeping tablets were conducted almost exclusively among young adults (usually males) despite the fact that the bulk of all sleeping tablets are prescribed for and consumed by middle-aged and elderly adults (usually females). The reasons for this anomaly are easily identified, but perhaps less easily excused. Sleep laboratories tend to be situated in colleges, universities, or medical schools. When preparing an experiment, therefore, researchers have generally found it easiest to recruit human subjects from the readily available student population. This predilection for young students has been greatly reinforced by the realisation among researchers that selecting older people for experiments requires more attention, effort, and time, than selecting young people. To understand why this should be the case, we need to consider some relevant aspects of experimental methodology, a detour which will also serve to highlight some interesting theoretical issues of importance in later chapters.

Most experiments involving animal subjects are not concerned with individual performance. There are some important exceptions but as a rule, groups of humans (or rats, or flatworms) are assembled by the investigator and each individual (human, rat, or flatworm) is measured on some characteristic of interest. The arithmetical average of these measurements, the mean, is then taken as representative of the whole group. Individuals show a sometimes quite irritating tendency to differ, and the degree to which a given mean value adequately represents a group will be greatly influenced by the degree of variability *within* the group. In particular, some members of a group may differ enormously from the rest and distort any information presented in average values. The mean age within a pre-school nursery class, for example, might be given as ten years old; the misleading consequence of including nine children of four years old and one teacher of 64 years old in the calculation. Not surprisingly, then, researchers take steps to reduce variability to a minimum within experimental groups, and to exclude possible statistical 'deviants'.

If the rules of random selection are observed, and all other things are equal, individuals within a group of young adults will be fairly evenly distributed above and below the mean value for most biologically determined characteristics (e.g. height, weight, total sleep time, number of awakenings during the night, etc.). Many of these characteristics will change with age. The problem for experimenters is that people do not age at the same rate; age-related changes occur rapidly in some individuals, and relatively slowly in others. Indeed, different organs and systems within the same body may age at different rates. The consequence of these differential rates of ageing is to increase variability among older people of the same age. At the age of 20, most people are physically healthy and active. At the age of 60, some will continue to be healthy and vigorous, some will be overweight and demonstrably inactive, and some will be physically impaired following heart attacks and other degenerative conditions. With passing time, chronological age becomes an increasingly imperfect predictor of ability and function, making 'the elderly' a very difficult group about which to make generalisations. Variability in the characteristics of groups of older subjects can be reduced to a minimum by careful screening, selectively removing, or only including, persons with certain illnesses or disabilities. This, however, is what requires attention, effort, and time and for many years researchers chose not to go to such lengths unless they were quite specifically interested in older sleep. If, on the other hand, they were interested in the effects of sleeping drugs, or alcohol, or exercise, or stress, or REM deprivation, or jet-lag, or numerous other influences upon sleep, then healthy young male adults were preferred.

In sleep research, as in many other branches of behavioural and biological science, interest in the elderly has grown rapidly in the last decade or so, and many of the methodological issues and problems which previously daunted investigators have been confronted and overcome. In the academic journal *Sleep Research* for the year 1974 only one report is indexed under the keyword 'elderly'. Five years later in 1979 there were eight such reports while in 1984 a total of 27 were listed. Throughout this period the total volume of sleep research, as indicated by published work, remained roughly constant. This shift in the priorities of sleep research may, at least in part, reflect increasing maturity among the first generation of EEG sleep researchers. In recent years, however, much of the increased scientific interest shown in the elderly has been provoked by demographic changes in both the number and the relative proportion of individuals reaching retirement and old age in the developed industrialised nations. In Great Britain, for example, the number of individuals aged 65 years and over rose from 5.3 million in 1951[14,15] to almost 8.0 million in 1981.[16] As proportions of the general population, these figures represent a rise from 11 per cent in 1951 to 15 per cent in 1981. In passing, it is interesting to note that this growth in the relative size of the elderly population is mainly the result not as is frequently supposed of medical technology increasing the average lifespan, but of fertility levels in the late nineteenth and early twentieth centuries.[17] In common with many other scientific disciplines, then, sleep research has responded, both metaphorically and literally, to market forces.

NOTES AND REFERENCES

1. Pavlov summarised his views on the control of sleep in a lecture given in Leningrad in December 1935, a transcript of which appears in: J. Gibbons, *I.P. Pavlov Selected Works* (translated by S. Belsky), Foreign Languages Publishing House, Moscow (1955). See especially the discussion on p. 386
2. This apparatus is fully described in N. Kleitman, *Sleep and*

Wakefulness, University of Chicago Press, Chicago, Chapter 10 (1963) pp. 81–91

3. See Mary A.B. Brazier, *A History of the Electrical Activity of the Brain: the First Half Century*, Pitman Medical Publishing Company Limited, London (1961)

4. A.L. Loomis, E.N. Harvey and G.A. Hobart, 'Electrical Potentials of the Human Brain', *Science*, 81 (1935) pp. 597–8

5. A.L. Loomis, E.N. Harvey and G.A. Hobart, 'Further Observations on the Potential Rhythms of the Cerebral Cortex During Sleep', *Science*, 82 (1935) pp. 198–200

6. E. Aserinsky and N. Kleitman, 'Regularly Occurring Periods of Eye Motility, and Concomitant Phenomena During Sleep', *Science*, 118 (1953) pp. 273–4

7. R.J. Berger, 'Tonus of Extrinsic Laryngeal Muscles During Sleep and Dreaming', *Science*, 134 (1961) p. 840

8. A. Rechtschaffen and A. Kales, *A Manual of Standardized Terminology, Techniques, and Scoring System for Sleep Stages of Human Subjects*, National Institute of Health Publication No. 24, Government Printing Office, Washington D.C. (1968)

9. G.T. Fechner, *Elemente der Psychophysik* (1860) English translation by D.H. Howes and E.G. Boring, *Elements of Psychophysics*, Chicago (1966)

10. See, for example P.A. Parish, 'The Prescribing of Psychotropic Drugs in General Practice', *Journal of the Royal College of General Practitioners*, Supplement No. 4, 21 (1971)

11. These and other methods are described in I. Oswald, 'Sleep Studies in Clinical Pharmacology', *British Journal of Clinical Pharmacology*, 10 (1980) pp. 317–26

12. This particular example comes from H.P. Roffwarg, J.N. Muzio, and W.C. Dement, 'Ontogenetic Development of the Human Sleep-Dream Cycle', *Science*, 152 (1966) pp. 604–19

13. See M.A. Carskadon, E.D. Brown and W.C. Dement, 'Sleep Fragmentation in the Elderly: Relationship to Daytime Sleep Tendency', *Neurobiology of Aging*, 3 (1982) pp. 321–7, for a full description of this procedure

14. General Register Office, *Census 1951 (England and Wales)*, Preliminary Report, HMSO, London (1956)

15. General Register Office Edinburgh, *Census 1951 (Scotland)*, General Volume, HMSO, Edinburgh (1954)

16. Office of Population Censuses and Surveys and Registrar General Scotland, *Census 1981 (Great Britain) Persons of Pensionable Age*, HMSO, London (1983)

17. The arguments supporting this conclusion are clearly summarised by E. Garfield, 'Social Gerontology. Part 2. Demography. The effects of an Ageing Population on Society', *Current Contents* (22) 28 (May 1984)

2

Sleep: Typical Age-related Changes

The likelihood of change occurring in previously well-established sleeping patterns increases with age. Some of these changes may be short-lived, while others may become stable features of our day-to-day and night-to-night lives. Advancing age is also associated with a steadily increasing variety of unwelcome events which can impinge upon and disrupt our sleep. Some of these events are transient and one-off, while others may recur throughout later life. In this and the following chapter age-related influences on sleep will be described and, with the help of examples selected from the research literature, their impact upon older people's sleep will be assessed. In order to structure and clarify this discussion, I will first consider, in very general terms, ways in which the process of ageing can affect sleep.

As outlined in Figure 2.1, the ageing process can influence sleep either directly or indirectly. Directly influenced changes are those which are due, or are assumed to be due to the ageing of the nervous system and the physiological mechanisms which control sleep and waking. An example of such directly influenced change is the progressive decline in the amount of stage 4 (slow wave) sleep throughout early and late adulthood. In so far as they occur in ostensibly healthy individuals and are not associated with any known disease process, directly influenced changes can be considered normal. Events which can affect sleep indirectly are those which arise outside of the physiological 'sleep system'[1] but, by impinging upon it, can profoundly affect the distribution and the structure of sleep. As shown in Figure 2.1, these events can be further divided into those which originate in the physical environment (mainly inside the body) and those which originate in the social

Figure 2.1: How ageing can influence sleep

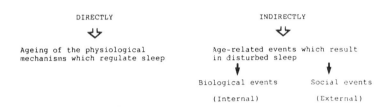

environment (mainly outside the body). Indirect influences from the physical environment include disruptions of sleep due to discomforting or painful diseases, and disruptions due to apparently normal senescent changes in those physiological systems not directly related to the control of sleep. The joint pains of osteoarthritis provide an example of the former, while night-time visits to the bathroom due to the ageing of mechanisms controlling bladder function illustrates the latter.

Ageing also has a social dimension and in addition to the essentially biological events so far considered, many of the social consequences of ageing can also interfere with sleep. Examples from this large category of disruptive influences include the emotional distress of bereavement, or the physical distress of a cold bedroom inadequately heated because of poverty. Other effects of 'social' (as opposed to biological) ageing on sleep may be a little more oblique. For example, it has long been evident from laboratory studies that unfamiliar surroundings and enforced departures from daily routine disturb sleep at least for the first night or so. (For this reason it is a common research practice to disregard the first and sometimes also the second night's EEG recordings and use only recordings made on subsequent consecutive visits to the laboratory when sleep patterns have settled down.) With advancing age the likelihood of being transferred or admitted to new and unfamiliar surroundings like hospitals, nursing homes, sheltered housing, or residential old-people's homes, etc. steadily increases, and the consequent likelihood of disturbed sleep, also increases.

Finally, it should be noted that the descriptive categories shown in Figure 2.1 are not mutually exclusive; disruptive influences upon sleep are, at any age, potentially additive and events from one category can, and in old age frequently do combine with events from another. Furthermore, the categories themselves are not perfectly distinct and to some extent overlap. With these imperfections in mind, the direct influence of ageing upon sleep will be considered in the present chapter while the indirect influence of ageing upon sleep will be discussed in Chapter 3.

CHANGES IN SLEEP DIRECTLY INFLUENCED BY THE AGEING PROCESS

Subjective quality of sleep

Deteriorating sleep quality has long been recognised as a feature of the ageing process, and sleeplessness has not infrequently been included among the more traditionally listed maladies of old age. In 1842 at the age of 71, for example, the essayist and cleric Sydney Smith wrote 'We are, at the close of life, only hurried away from stomach aches, pains in the joints, from sleepless nights and unamusing days'.[2] Similar associations between ageing and sleep were noted by the novelist Herman Melville who in 1851 both acknowledged and rather drily explained the sleeplessness of old age as follows: 'Old age is always wakeful; as if, the longer linked with life, the less man has to do with aught that looks like death'.[3] Clinical attention to the topic has a similarly long history and allusions to age-related sleep problems are not uncommon in early nineteenth century medical journals. Writing in the *The Lancet* in 1836 Dr George Sigmond of the Windmill Street School of Medicine, London, summarised his impressions of changing sleep patterns thus: 'The duration of sleep should be, in manhood, about the fourth or the sixth of the 24 hours; children, the younger they are the more sleep they require; in advanced age there is more watchfulness [sleeplessness]'.[4] While Dr Sigmond's expectation of average sleep length in nineteenth century manhood does seem a little unrealistic (a mere 4-6 hours) he nevertheless succinctly identifies a relationship between increasing age and decreasing quality of sleep.

In recent years links between ageing and declining sleep quality have been confirmed in questionnaire surveys conducted

Figure 2.2: Percentage of people in different age groups reporting 'frequent' night-time awakenings; results from a survey of 2446 people living in Scotland

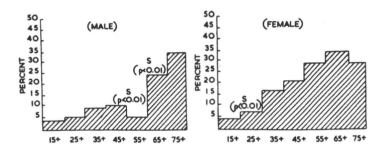

Note: Where differences between men and women are greater than expected by chance alone, this is indicated by the symbol 'S'.
Source: McGhie and Russell (1962) 'The Subjective Assessment of Normal Sleep Patterns', *Journal of Mental Science*, Vol. 108 (1962) pp. 642–54. Reprinted with permission.

both in Britain and in the United States. One of the first major studies of this kind, reported by doctors Andrew McGhie and S.M. Russell in 1962, analysed the subjective sleep characteristics of 2446 individuals of all ages living in the Dundee and Glasgow areas of Scotland.[5] These researchers found a clear relationship between age and subjective appraisals of certain aspects of sleep. Specifically, increasing age was associated with a greater likelihood of reporting frequent night awakenings (see Figure 2.2) and early morning awakening. Furthermore, when asked to rate their sleep as 'deep', 'moderate', or 'light', older people were more likely to describe themselves as light sleepers. Some 16 years later Dr Ismet Karacan and colleagues working at the University of Florida, USA, found very similar age-related sleep characteristics in the questionnaire responses of 1645 individuals living in Alachua County in north-central Florida.[6] In answer to the rather general question 'How often do you have trouble sleeping?', the proportion of individuals responding 'sometimes' or 'often or all the time' increased steadily with age (see Figure 2.3). For the age group 70 years and over, almost 26 per cent reported having trouble with their sleep at least 'often', compared with only 6.2 per cent of those aged 19

Figure 2.3: Percentage of people in different age groups reporting 'trouble with sleeping'; results from a survey of 1645 people living in Florida, USA

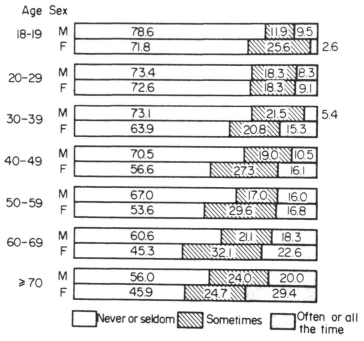

Source: Karacan *et al.*, 'Prevalence of Sleep Disturbance in a Primarily Urban Florida County' *Social Science and Medicine,* Vol. 10 (1976) pp. 239–44. Reprinted with permission.

years and under. When individuals were asked to specify what *kind* of trouble they had, complaints of difficulty in staying asleep, and of early morning awakening tended, as in the Scottish study, to be more frequent with increasing age. Clearly, age-related dissatisfaction with sleep shows considerable concordance between cultures and, if comparing Scotland and Florida, between climates. Both surveys show agreement on three complaints in relation to age; older sleep is experienced as shorter, lighter, and more broken. Both surveys also showed that, from early adulthood to old age, women are more likely to report dissatisfaction with their sleep than are men, an issue to which we shall return in Chapter 4.

In contrast to *staying* asleep, *getting* to sleep is less frequently reported as a problem by older people. In two British surveys, one conducted in Camden, London by Dr P. Gerard and colleagues,[7] and the other conducted in Huddersfield, Yorkshire by Ken Gledhill,[8] complaints of disturbed sleep were found to be 2 – 3 times more likely than complaints of getting to sleep among elderly individuals. Nevertheless, age-related dissatis-faction with the efficiency of sleep onset should not be underrated. In a survey sponsored by the World Health Organization[9] and conducted in ten European countries and one middle-eastern country (Kuwait) in 1979, men and women aged from 60 – 89 were asked whether they had experienced any difficulty in falling asleep in the previous two weeks. From locations ranging from Finland to rural Greece, and from Normandy to Kiev reports of difficulty in falling asleep tended to increase steadily from the youngest to the oldest group. Unfortunately, questions about staying asleep were not included in this survey providing, perhaps, further evidence of the wide-spread failure to appreciate the changing characteristics of sleep that go with advancing age, even amongst those who should know better.

The decreasing satisfaction with sleep found among older individuals can, of course, be interpreted in different ways. Rather than indicating actual changes in sleep, such dissatisfaction may reflect little more than an age-related propensity for complaining! How, then, do these subjective reports relate to objective (polysomnographic) measurements of sleep? The answer to this question has emerged from laboratory studies which, over the past 20 years, have been concerned with establishing age-related electroencephalographic 'norms' of human sleep in relation to age. In practice, this has been accomplished either by recording the sleep of many different age groups or, more simply and more cheaply by comparing the sleep recordings obtained from a single group of older volunteers with those obtained from a group of younger volunteers. Examples from both of these approaches will be presented in the discussion which follows.

EEG characteristics of sleep

Sleep stage profiles typical of healthy young and elderly individuals are shown in Figure 2.4. By comparing Figures 2.4(a) and 2.4(b) it can be seen that older sleep shows structural

Figure 2.4(a) and 2.4(b): Typical hypnogram for young adults (above) and for the elderly (below)

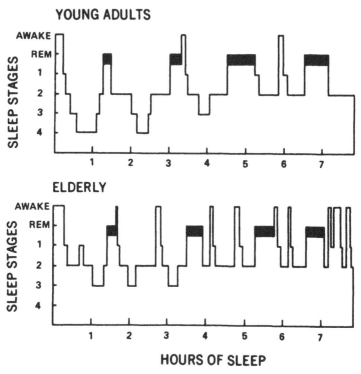

Source: Kales *et al.*, UCLA Interdepartmental Conference on Sleep and Dreams, *Annals of Internal Medicine*, Vol. 68 (1968) pp. 1078–104. Reprinted with permission.

changes consistent with the subjective complaints already described. Compared with that of young adults, the sleep profile for the elderly appears more broken, less deep and, in terms of the actual time spent asleep, shorter. Like the transition from youth to old age the transition from young sleep to old sleep is not abrupt. Contributing to the latter profile are gradual changes in many of the characteristics of sleep measured by the EEG. To assess the impact of ageing on different aspects of sleep, each of these characteristics will be considered in the order in which they were defined in Table 1.1.

Sleep onset latency. In 1959 work commenced at the University of Florida under the direction of Dr R.L. Williams which, 13 years and several thousands of miles of EEG traces later produced sleep-stage information on eleven different age groups ranging from 3 – 5 year olds (Group 1) to 70 – 79 year olds (Group 11).[10] This programme of research found little change in the time taken to fall asleep between the ages of 3 and 69 in males, and 3 and 79 in females. Across these age groups the average latency ranged from only 6 to 20 minutes with the longest average latencies of about 18.5 minutes associated with females aged 10 – 12 and 16 – 19. The males aged over 70, however, appeared to have most difficulty in falling asleep; while the average latency for this group was 32 minutes, at least one member of the group remained awake for almost an hour before falling asleep. As pointed out in the previous chapter, such extreme fluctuations within a group become increasingly common as the age of the group increases and should be taken into account when interpreting average values. Ageing individuals do not change at the same rate and, as regards sleep, some individuals hardly change at all.

It is relevant to note here that the actual number of people within each of the eleven age groups used in the Florida studies was relatively small, never less than ten but no more than 13, a feature which may limit the representativeness of the information reported. Nevertheless other research workers have reported very similar sleep latencies in larger groups of older subjects. Among 40 male and 40 female volunteers aged between 50 and 60 years, Dr Wilse B. Webb, also of the University of Florida, found average sleep onset latencies of 12.7 minutes for the men and 17.6 minutes for the women.[11] Similar sleep latencies are also reported by Dr Irwin Feinberg who, in his pioneering research into the sleep patterns of the very elderly, found that the average time taken to fall asleep in six women and nine men aged between 65 and 96 years was 18.5 minutes.[12]

Sleep period time. The sleep period – the time from sleep onset to final awakening – shows little consistent change with advancing age. Among the subjects aged between 40 – 79 studied by the Florida group, the average sleep period time rose from 432.3 minutes to 470.7 minutes for women, and from 419.9 minutes to 448.8 minutes for men. Once again, however, variability within groups increased substantially with age and

Figure 2.5: Average (mean) frequency of night-time awakenings recorded in eleven age groups

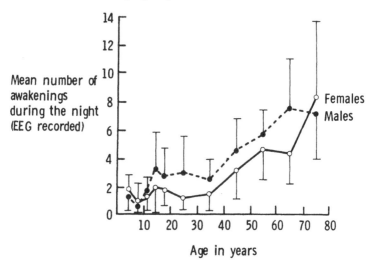

Each point represents the average for at least 10 subjects

Note: Vertical lines indicate the standard deviation from the mean within each age group.
Source: From Williams *et al., EEG of Human Sleep: Clinical Applications,* New York, Wiley (1974). Reprinted with permission.

some individuals showed little or no change in their sleep period. As will be seen below, an increase in the sleep period time by no means indicates an increase in actual total sleep.

Intervening wakefulness. While sleep latency and sleep period show only slight and rather inconsistent changes, both the frequency and the total duration of wakefulness after sleep onset increase steadily with advancing age. Figure 2.5 shows the average number of awakenings during sleep for each of the eleven age groups in the Florida programme, while Figure 2.4(b) indicates the typical distribution of such awakenings throughout the night. The number of awakenings shows a clear tendency to increase for both sexes after the age of 40, with another steep increase for females after the age of 60, these periods of wakefulness tending to cluster in the latter half of the night (see Figure 2.4(b)). It can also be seen from Figure 2.5

that from shortly after the age of puberty until well into the sixth decade of life, males tend to wake more frequently than females. Dr Williams and his co-authors have speculated that this difference between the sexes may be due to the disturbing effects of penile erections which, as mentioned in Chapter 1, occur quite mechanically during REM sleep.

The research evidence also shows that the duration of each of these episodes of intervening wakefulness tends to increase with age, suggesting that older individuals not only wake more frequently during the night, but also experience greater difficulty in returning to sleep once disturbed. Combining all episodes of sleep stage 0 (wakefulness) with stage 1 (drowsiness) Dr Vlasta Brezinova working at the University Department of Psychiatry in Edinburgh, found a higher proportion of prolonged episodes of '0+1' in 14 older subjects aged 42 – 66 than in ten younger subjects aged 20 – 30.[13] Similarly, in the study by W.B. Webb mentioned above, the longest period of wakefulness for males and females in the 50 – 60 age group was 17.1 and 12.3 minutes respectively compared with 2.8 minutes for the males and 3.1 minutes for the females in the younger group. The combined effect of the more frequent occurrence and the longer duration of intervening wakefulness is, of course, to greatly increase the total amount of time spent awake during the sleep period. In the Florida study, for example, the total duration of wakefulness after sleep onset between the ages of 20 – 79 increased from just over two minutes to over 57 minutes for women, and from just over five minutes to 76 minutes for men. Other studies have reported increases of a similar order. Clearly, sleep in the older person is more fragmented or broken.

Stage shifts. The number of shifts or transitions from one sleep stage to another (including shifts into wakefulness) also shows a progressive age-related increase. This trend is clearly shown in Figure 2.4 ((a) and (b)), each vertical line of the profiles representing one shift. It can also be seen from this figure that the increased number of shifts in old age results not only from the increased frequency of awakening, but also from an increased number of brief episodes of stage 1 sleep (drowsiness). As the experience of broken or restless sleep is known to be associated with an increase in EEG stage shifts, Figure 2.4(b) accords well with the quality of sleep reported by many elderly

29

Figure 2.6: Changes with age in daily amounts of total sleep.

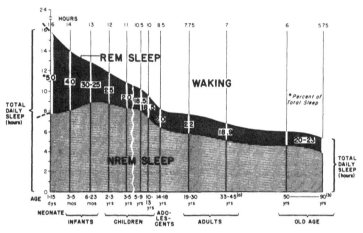

REM SLEEP/NREM SLEEP RELATIONSHIP
THROUGHOUT HUMAN LIFE

Note the sharp diminution of REM sleep in the early years. REM sleep falls from eight hours at birth to less than one hour in old age. The amount of non-REM (NREM) sleep throughout life remains more constant, falling from eight hours to five hours. In contrast to the steep decline of REM sleep, the quantity of NREM sleep is undiminished for many years. Although total daily REM sleep falls steadily during life, the percentage rises slightly in adolescence and early adulthood. This rise does not reflect an increase in amount; it is due to the fact that REM sleep does not diminish as quickly as total sleep. Data for the 33 – 45 and 50 – 90 year groups taken from Kales *et al.* (1967), Feinberg *et al.* (1967), and Kahn and Fisher (1969).
Source: Revised by Roffwarg *et al.* since publication in *Science*, Vol. 152 (1966) pp. 604–19. Reprinted with permission.

individuals. There are incidentally 26 shifts shown in Figure 2.4(a), compared with 42 in Figure 2.4(b).

Total sleep time. As periods of intervening wakefulness increase in frequency and duration with age, total sleep time shows a reciprocal decrease. Information published by Dr Howard P. Roffwarg and colleagues in 1966[14] and since updated as shown in Figure 2 6, illustrates the relative speed with which total sleep time decreases. The decrease goes from an average of 16 hours per day in 1 – 15 day old infants, to an average of only 5.75 hours per day at the age of 90. While the rate of change is undoubtedly most rapid in infancy and adolescence total sleep time maintains a steady decline from young adulthood to old age. Again it should be emphasised that variability among individuals also increases with age and that extreme deviations from these average times are relatively more common in the elderly.

Duration of each sleep stage. Both REM and NREM sleep show a proportionate decline with advancing age such that their relative share of total sleep time remains fairly constant throughout adult life. From the various studies contributing to Figure 2.6, for example, it can be seen that for the groups of people aged 14 – 19 and 50 – 90 years, stage REM averages about 20 per cent of the time spent asleep. A consequence of this reduction in the *absolute* duration of REM, and one that will be considered in the final chapter, is to reduce the opportunities for vivid dreaming in older persons. (It should not be assumed from this, however, that dreaming occurs *only* during REM sleep. As Dr Roffwarg and colleagues point out 'ideational material and poorly defined imagery can apparently persist throughout the entire range of sleep stages'. Nevertheless, the most vividly recalled dreams tend to be associated with the REM periods.)[14] One of the most consistently reported age-related changes in NREM sleep is the progressive reduction in EEG slow waves (those associated with stages 3 and 4 or 'deep' sleep) and, in many older individuals, the virtual disappearance of stage 4 altogether. Indeed, many researchers omit the distinction between stages 3 and 4 in older volunteers and simply aggregate all slow wave sleep into a single category of 'stage 3 + 4'. In the Florida studies none of the men, and only four of the ten women in the age group 70 – 79 years exhibited stage 4 sleep. Expressed as percentages of the sleep period time both stage 3 and stage 2 show a tendency first to increase and then decrease with advancing age. While changes in stage 2 show little overall difference between the sexes, the Florida studies found that with advancing age men have increasingly less stage 3 than women. As suggested by the results from Dr Brezinova's study, the relative contribution of stage 1 sleep (drowsiness) to the sleep period time increases steadily through-out life but, as is again evident from the Florida studies, men tend to have a higher percentage of stage 1 sleep than females from puberty onwards. Nevertheless, the age-related changes in sleep structure considered in this section result in lighter more easily disturbed sleep for both sexes.

Time in bed. It is paradoxical that although actual sleep time diminishes with age the total amount of time spent in bed per night appears to increase from middle age onwards. When allowed to 'free run' (i.e. arise at will) Dr Williams and his colleagues at the University of Florida found that time in bed rose from 441.5 minutes and 429.1 minutes respectively for women and men aged between 40 – 49 years, to 507.1 and 493.1 minutes for women and men aged 70 – 79 years (an increase of over one hour for both sexes). Nor is this an isolated finding. In the previously mentioned study conducted in New York by Irwin Feinberg and colleagues, healthy elderly volunteers spent, on average, over 48 minutes longer in bed than younger individuals aged from 19 to 36 even though both groups could remain in bed 'according to individual preference'. One possible explanation for this behaviour is that older people attempt to make up for sleep lost during the night by staying in bed longer in the morning.

Sleep efficiency. The combined result of decreasing sleep time and increasing time in bed is to greatly decrease the value of the sleep efficiency index (i.e. total sleep time divided by the total time spent in bed). For males and females aged 20 – 29 years, the Florida group report sleep efficiency indexes of 0.95 and 0.96 respectively. For males and females in the age group 70 – 79 years however, the values are 0.77 and 0.82 respectively. Assuming that the primary purpose of being in bed is to sleep, then a sleep efficiency index of one is equivalent to perfect sleep, while lower values of this index reflect increasing degrees of sleeplessness or sleep 'inefficiency'.

In general age-related complaints about the quality and quantity of sleep, as found in population surveys, are consistent with the structural changes in sleep found in laboratory studies. Since the pioneering studies of Feinberg, Williams, Webb and their colleagues, portable polysomnographs accompanied by mobile sleep researchers have confirmed these laboratory findings in the comfort of the subject's own homes.[15] At home or in the laboratory the sleep of the older person appears, and is experienced as, lighter, more broken, and shorter.

Depth of sleep

Inevitably, a reduction in slow wave sleep and a reciprocal increase in the lighter stage 1, greatly reduces the overall depth of sleep in older individuals. Nevertheless, the lightening of sleep with age is not only due to these structural changes. In addition to profound reductions in deep sleep and reciprocal increases in drowsiness and wakefulness, individual sleep stages themselves become lighter and more easily disturbed with increasing age. As described in Chapter 1, depth of sleep can be expressed in terms of the minimum amount of noise required to wake the sleeping individual — the auditory arousal or auditory awakening threshold. In a study conducted by Dr Harold Zepelin and his colleagues at Oakland University in the United States, the auditory awakening thresholds for men and women in three age groups (18 – 24, 40 – 48, and 52 – 71) were assessed by playing recordings of five second tones into hearing aids worn by these sleeping volunteers.[16] Tones were repeated, each louder than the last, until the volunteer awoke and pushed a button attached to the bed. The results from this procedure clearly show that during stages 2, 4 and REM, the amount of noise pressure (measured in decibels) required to waken the sleeping subjects declined with age for both men and women. In each of these sleep stages, then, the older individuals were more easily awakened by noise, despite the fact that younger individuals have more sensitive hearing both in this study and in general.

Under normal circumstances, however, the chances of being exposed to an intermittent electronic tone which slowly and relentlessly increases in volume until it disturbs our sleep may be remote. More typical of the sounds likely to disturb sleep are sudden loud noises (bumps and bangs) or rapid crescendos (a passing motor cycle or aeroplane, for example). The effects on sleep of this type of noise have been extensively studied by Jerome Lukas at the Sensory Sciences Research Center in California who has found that the sleep of older individuals is much more likely to be disturbed by simulated sonic booms than is the sleep of younger people.[17] Furthermore, Lukas also reports that when exposed to simulated aircraft flyover noises or simulated sonic booms middle aged women were more likely than middle aged men to be disturbed in their sleep. It would be reasonable to conclude, therefore, that with increasing age sleep becomes more sensitive to the disruptive influence of noise and that, under some circumstances, this sensitivity is greatest in females. Unfortunately, studies employing a realism somewhere between electronic tones and simulated sonic booms are relatively scarce, and little direct research has been conducted into the effects of environmental noise on the sleep of the elderly in the community. Indirect evidence does suggest that an age-related sensitivity to things that go bump in the night is not uncommon. In a major survey of mental health problems among elderly citizens randomly selected from the populations of London and New York, 3 per cent of those questioned in both cities reported noise as a specific problem for sleeping. This happened even though 28 per cent of New Yorkers and 38 per cent of Londoners claimed to have hearing difficulties![18] (Further results from this study, reported by Dr Barry Gurland and his colleagues will be considered in more detail in Chapter 3.)

Daytime napping

Age-related changes in sleeping patterns are not confined to the night-time. A further almost stereotypic feature of advancing age is an increasing tendency to nap during the day. In conjunction with those changes in night-time sleep already considered, daytime napping can be viewed as a redistribution of sleep across the 24 hour period. Indeed, it has frequently been suggested that the slowly alternating, biphasic sleep–wake rhythm of the adult begins in old age to resemble the rapidly alternating *multiphasic* sleep–wake rhythm of the young child. In addition to reinforcing a rather cosy stereotyped image of the elderly (the image which accompanies the ill-advised 'well earned rest' in retirement, for instance) daytime naps can help to throw some light on the nature of changing patterns of sleep seen in the elderly. Surprisingly, however, survey information on the extent to which elderly individuals are likely to engage in daytime napping, or the average duration of such naps is a bit patchy and sometimes inconsistent. Of the 2,446 individuals of all ages who completed the sleep questionnaire in McGhie and Russell's Scottish survey,[5] only 42 (1.7 per cent) reported taking a daytime nap, a finding which suggests that napping during the day is not a particularly common practice. However, in the survey of sleep patterns in the elderly conducted in Camden, London, and briefly mentioned above, over half of the 55 young and nearly two-thirds of the 103 elderly adults who returned questionnaires admitted that, in recent months, they had dozed or slept during the day.[7]

As is always the case when comparing questionnaire studies, different responses to apparently similar questions may be due to the way in which the questions were phrased. In the Camden survey, the question referred to naps taken 'over recent months', while it appears that the Scottish survey asked whether the respondent 'usually' napped or slept during the day. In the sleep survey conducted in Huddersfield, Yorkshire, Gledhill[8] found that out of 109 elderly people living in sheltered housing, or attending a day centre, 42 per cent reported that they had taken a nap on the previous day — a proportion much closer to that found in London. In addition to differences in the way questions are phrased, other reasons might also influence people's responses to questions on napping. It should be remembered, for example, that sleeping during the day is not entirely unconnected with a social image of sloth and laziness, and that some individuals may simply prefer not to admit to it, especially in those cultures where the work ethic is particularly strong. Reports of daytime napping also show some interesting differences between the sexes. Questionnaires completed by the 40 male and 40 female participants in Dr W.B. Webb's previously mentioned sleep study revealed that while over 70 per cent of men and women admitted to sleeping in the daytime, these naps were more frequent, though shorter, in the men.[11]

More detailed, and more accurate, analyses of daytime napping are provided by studies in which the sleeping and waking behaviour of elderly individuals has either been observed or instrumentally measured throughout the 24 hour day. A rather gruelling study in which the behaviour of 19 elderly inpatients 'with only the general debilities of aging' was observed and recorded every 15 minutes during two 36 hour periods was reported by Wilse B. Webb and Heather Swinburne in 1971 while Dr Webb was a visiting lecturer at the University of Cambridge.[19] Only one of the observed patients failed to take a daytime nap in the 72 hours of observation. Of the remainder, the 9 men took an average of 1.8 naps per day, while the 10 women took an average of 1.4 naps per day. As might be expected, individuals varied greatly, some spending three or more periods asleep during the daytime. In this study naps tended to occur rather haphazardly throughout the day and, although observations were obtained for four separate daytime periods (the 36 hour period extended from 8 a.m. on the first day to 8 p.m. on the second day), no consistent 'pattern' of daytime napping emerged. From the evidence considered so far, napping does appear to be fairly common among the elderly living in the community, and extremely common among the more dependent elderly living in institutions.

As with night-time sleep, the most accurate way to quantify daytime naps is to use either the EEG or an instrumental measurement closely related to the EEG. Sleep laboratories, however, tend to be rather impersonal high-tech bedrooms without the facilities for comfortable daytime recording, let alone comfortable daytime naps. On the other hand, home recordings made in a more natural environment using less intrusive apparatus offer an ideal opportunity for studying episodes of sleep taken out of bed. Using lightweight equipment which records breathing, leg-muscle tension, and wrist movement, an extensive programme of home sleep recordings of the elderly was conducted in San Diego, California by Dr Sonia Ancoli-Israel and her collaborators.[20] (When compared with the EEG, such recordings are quite good at distinguishing between sleep and wakefulness.) While the main purpose of this study was to identify breathing difficulties and body movements during sleep, the method of recording does provide some insights into the frequency and duration of daytime naps. Each volunteer was connected to the recording apparatus at about 6 p.m., and disconnected the following day at about 8.30 a.m.

In this way an average of about 14.5 hours of recording was obtained from 145 randomly selected volunteers aged between 65 and 95 years. Each of these subjects also maintained a diary in which they recorded their bedtime and their time of getting up. When the recordings and the diary entries were compared it was found that 94 per cent of the volunteers had taken a nap either shortly before their reported bedtime or soon after their reported getting up time. In fact, 91 per cent of all napping occurred within one hour of going to or getting out of bed, with the average time spent in naps being 59.7 minutes in the evening, and 32.3 minutes in the morning. Evidently, many of these elderly individuals fell asleep in the late evening, woke up and decided it was time for bed. From questionnaire surveys and instrumental home recordings it would appear that napping is a fairly common characteristic among older people.

Daytime napping and night-time sleep

Why, then, do older people nap? Theoretically, napping in older people can be related to at least three causal factors. First, in much the same way as a younger individual they may nap in order to compensate for sleep lost or degraded during the previous night. Second, because of changes in the external social structure, napping in older people may result from understimulation and perhaps a weakening of the social constraints which usually discourage such behaviours in younger individuals, such as loss of employment. Third, older people may nap because the biological clock which regulates the circadian rhythm of sleep and wakefulness in adults is showing signs of wear and tear and, as mentioned earlier, the biphasic sleep-wake cycle may be giving way to the multiphasic rhythms characteristic of young children. For each of these propositions the implications for night-time sleep are rather different. It has been suggested, for example, that the reduction of total sleep time with increasing age may represent a diminishing need for sleep in older individuals.[21] If, however, daytime naps are an attempt to compensate for lost night-time sleep, then suggestions of a reduced sleep need become less plausible. On the other hand, if naps are principally the consequence of understimulation and daytime routines lacking in structure, then it is possible that they are a contributing cause rather than the direct effect of poor night-time sleep. After all, habitual daytime napping cannot but influence the character of night-time sleep.

The third proposition, an age-related decline in the efficiency of the circadian clock mediating sleep and wakefulness, offers a simultaneous explanation for both increased daytime and decreased night-time sleep. Thus, rather than one of these events causing the other, they may have a common cause. Logically, there is absolutely nothing preventing all three of these explanations and others besides combining and, in the same individual, contributing to the sleep–wake patterns observed in many elderly people. Nevertheless, the available evidence does allow for the likely contribution of each of these factors to be assessed. A discussion of daytime napping also provides an opportunity to consider some of the daytime consequences of age-related changes in adult sleep.

Tiredness and sleepiness during the day. Some of the earliest experiments ever conducted in sleep research were concerned with the effects of sleep deprivation. This interesting line of inquiry was, in fact, based upon a principle that has for many years been frequently and profitably applied in biological science: if you want to discover the function of an organ, remove it and observe the consequences. In much the same way, sleep deprivation was seen as a way of learning about the function or purpose of sleep, and numerous tests were employed to measure the possible psychological consequences of prolonged sleeplessness. Those consequences, however, were to prove rather difficult to detect. For example, measuring muscle strength, speed of reaction, or intellectual performance, researchers found that even after many hours of sleep deprivation individuals were just as strong, could be just as quick, and could respond just as intelligently as they had done when completely rested. On one thing all researchers agreed, the longer a person is kept awake the more that person will want to go to sleep. Deprivation of sleep makes people very tired. If sleep becomes more broken and shorter with increasing age, the possibility exists that older people become progressively sleep-deprived and that daytime napping is a normal and predictable consequence of this deprivation. As will be seen below, the research evidence does not wholly support this view.

The simplest way of addressing the issue of whether or not ageing adults typically suffer progressive sleep deprivation is to ask the question, 'Do older people feel more tired than younger people when they get out of bed?' From the Scottish survey of McGhie and Russell, the answer appears to be a clear 'No'. In fact, when asked if they usually felt tired in the morning, older people in this survey were *less* likely to say yes. Furthermore, in questionnaire studies that have attempted to relate reported quality of sleep in the elderly to reported daytime tiredness, no clear relationship has been found. In Gledhill's study of 109 elderly people in Yorkshire, for example, those who reported feelings of tiredness during the daytime were just as likely to have reported poor quality sleep as those who experienced little or no tiredness. In other words, reports of daytime tiredness in the elderly may be influenced by factors other than the amount or quality of sleep on the previous night (they might, for example, be influenced by mood).

Feelings of tiredness are closely related to the degree of daytime sleepiness. It will be recalled from Chapter 1 that, whereas 'tiredness' is a subjective, introspective description, 'sleepiness' can be measured simply as the time taken to fall asleep when lying comfortably in a darkened quiet room, the so-called daytime sleep tendency or sleep latency. Are elderly people more sleepy than younger people during the day? Using this technique to measure sleepiness in different age groups, Dr Mary Carskadon and her colleagues at Stanford University, California, have found that, in general, elderly people are sleepier during the day than young adults, who in turn are sleepier than children.[22] Nevertheless it cannot be assumed that older people are invariably more sleepy during the day. Results from the Stanford laboratory have shown that some healthy young people can fall asleep much faster than the 'average' elderly person.[23] The fact that no simple relationship exists between the characteristics of night-time sleep and the likely occurrence of daytime naps is illustrated by studies in which both sleep and subsequent sleepiness have been recorded in the same individuals. At the Stanford laboratory Dr Carskadon and others measured the night-time sleep and daytime sleep tendency in 24 elderly volunteers aged from 63 to 86.[24] Following a night in the laboratory during which sleep and breathing were recorded, the daytime sleep tendency of each volunteer was measured every two hours from 9.30 in the morning until 7.30 in the evening, a total of six measurements. At these times throughout the day the volunteers lay down in bed, closed their eyes, and tried to fall asleep while connected to the EEG machine. If the volunteer fell asleep within 20 minutes, then the sleep latency, that is, the time taken to fall asleep, provided the test score. If the volunteer failed to fall asleep in the allotted 20 minutes then the test was called off.

With the information collected in this study, the researchers were able to compare the structure of sleep recorded at night with the degree of sleepiness measured throughout the following day in each of these healthy subjects. Interestingly, the average daytime sleep latency, that is, average daytime sleepiness, was not related to the length of sleep on the previous night. Nor was sleepiness related to the number of awakenings after sleep onset, the number of stage shifts, the number of bodily movements, or the duration of any of the five sleep stages on the previous night. There did appear to be a relationship, however, between increased daytime sleepiness and the way in which the subject breathed during night-time sleep. Specifically, frequent episodes of shallow breathing or recurrent long delays between breaths were associated with shorter daytime sleep latencies. It was also found in this study that daytime sleepiness was related to the number of transient EEG arousals during the night. These rather curious arousals appear on the EEG trace as brief bursts of (usually) alpha activity lasting from 2 – 15 seconds which are not associated with awakening or with a change in the sleep stage, but are associated with the changes in the depth or frequency of breathing during sleep. Taken together these micro-disturbances seem to make a greater contribution to daytime sleepiness and perhaps daytime napping, than the more traditionally emphasised changes in older sleep like total sleep time or the number of awakenings during the night.

Nevertheless, these apparently influential disturbances of sleep by no means accounted for the degree of daytime sleepiness measured in all subjects, emphasising the absence of a straightforward one-to-one relationship between the characteristics of the sleep of the older person, and the propensity for taking naps during the day. Furthermore if, as seems to be the case, total sleep time is not the most important determinant of daytime sleep tendency in the elderly, then it cannot be assumed that by increasing night-time sleep the need for daytime naps will diminish. It is also of interest to note that, prior to taking part in Dr Carskadon's study, each of the 24 volunteers was asked to rate their own sleep. None reported feelings of daytime tiredness even though, from the results obtained, at least two were considered to have abnormally short daytime sleep latencies indicative of excessive daytime sleepiness. It will be remembered that the previously mentioned questionnaire surveys of sleep also showed low levels of reported tiredness. Perhaps for many elderly people the feelings accompanying an increased tendency to fall asleep when quiet and comfortable are experienced as qualitatively distinct from those associated with fatigue.

Do older people really sleep less? For many older adults sleep becomes a daily, as well as a nightly event. As we have seen, naps can occur in the morning, the afternoon, or the evening with perhaps some preference being shown for those taken later in the day. So far, however, we have only taken nocturnal sleep into account when calculating total sleep time. It is therefore reasonable to ask whether, if all periods of sleep throughout the 24 hours are taken into consideration, older people really do sleep less. Naturally, adding nap times to sleep times will reduce any differential between old and young sleepers, but it should be remembered that not all elderly people nap. In the study reported by Irwin Feinberg (the results from which contribute to the right hand tail of Figure 2.6), elderly volunteers were hospitalised for the few days of sleep recordings and 'special care' was taken 'to prevent the occurrence of daytime sleep'.[12] Even in the absence of napping, total sleep time was still reduced in the older volunteers. Habitual daytime napping was taken into consideration by Dr Patricia Prinz of the University of Washington who, in a series of studies of ageing sleep recorded the EEGs of twelve elderly people in their own homes.[15] Three of these were encouraged to take their habitual daytime naps which in each case exceeded one hour (the remaining nine were not habitual nappers). When these nap times were aggregated with sleep times, the average total sleep time for the group still remained lower than that for typical young adults. Other reports have indicated that, under some circumstances, older sleep times may equal or even exceed those of younger individuals (an example of the latter is Dr Webb's observational study of elderly hospital patients described earlier). Once again, it should be emphasised that people vary enormously in the degree to which, and the rate at which, they change with age. It cannot be stated as a general rule, therefore, that daytime napping entirely compensates for age-related reductions in nocturnal total sleep time. Many healthy, well adjusted individuals clearly sleep less as they grow older.

Naps as a response to tedium. At any age, a stimulating, challenging environment which commands our attention will promote vigilance and wakefulness, while boredom with or disinterest in what is going on around us promotes torpor and sleep. Even if we are thoroughly well rested from the night before monotonous events in which we play only a passive role can make us feel disinterested and sleepy. When the environment stops making demands upon us, or when we disengage from the environment, sleep becomes more probable. For most people who are engaged in formal employment, or for those with less formal but equally demanding responsibilities, daytime sleeping is neither practically nor socially encouraged. It might reasonably be supposed, however, that after the age of retirement many of the factors which previously operated to discourage daytime sleeping are removed or weakened. Life in old age may progressively become less complex and less demanding and, under such circumstances, daytime napping can emerge by default, that is, it might happen because nothing prevents it from happening. This, for example, appears to have been the case in the hospital where the daytime and night-time sleep behaviour of 19 elderly individuals was observed by Webb and Swinburne. At the end of their report they comment that 'The naps we have noted appeared to be somewhat random events unrelated to night sleep and often gave the impression of sheer boredom rather than an overwhelming "eruption" of sleep'.[19] Nevertheless, what dependent elderly people do in hospitals does not necessarily predict what healthy elderly people may do in their own homes.

A questionnaire survey conducted by Dr Zepelin of Oakland University, Michigan, among ex-college students reports information on napping which neither wholly supports, nor contradicts the supposition that daytime sleep in older people is frequently due to boredom.[25] From 469 responses to a postal questionnaire Dr Zepelin found that for men, daytime napping increased with age irrespective of employment status. Among women an age-related tendency to sleep during the day was present only among those not engaged in full time employment. (It may be assumed that a significant proportion of female ex-college students were professionally employed.) Thus, it would appear that even before retirement the habit of napping is already fairly well established among American professional males, while only among women was the absence of full time employment associated with an increase in daytime sleep. Once again, it is interesting to note this difference between the sexes which reinforces Webb and Swinburne's[19] earlier reported finding that men were more likely to take naps. The occurrence of napping among professional working men, however, is not entirely consistent with the idea that daytime sleeping is largely due to unstructured and tedious daily routines.

The redistribution of sleep. The alternating states of sleep and wakefulness are maintained by numerous physiological processes each roughly synchronised with the 24-hour day. These biological rhythms are not immutable and, if the external rhythms alter then, given sufficient time, the internal rhythms will adapt. These external rhythms are known as zeitgebers (a German word meaning 'timegiver'). Until the rhythm has adapted fully, however, it may be described as desynchronised. Jet lag is a typical example of desynchronisation, with the internal clock telling one time, and the external zeitgebers telling another. With advancing age it is likely that daytime napping and fragmented night-time sleep will contribute to the desynchronisation of a previously established sleep–wake cycle. There also exists the further possibility that age-related changes in the efficiency of the biological clock itself will result in, rather than be caused by, broken night-time sleep and daytime napping. It has been suggested, for example, that the normal sleep of some elderly people resembles the abnormal sleep of some regular transmeridian travellers, night-shift workers, and even some types of insomniac,[26] and that the pattern of broken night-time sleep, and periods of daytime sleepiness and napping seen in older people may result from chronic desynchronisation. At any age, events which can disturb synchronised sleep-wake routines are not uncommon. With advancing age, however, sleep appears to become less adaptable to changing circumstances with the result that older people are less able to take such events in their stride. That sleep does become less adaptable with increasing age is indicated by the response of older people to sleep disturbances incurred either experimentally, or quite naturally in the course of their work. Examples of both are provided below.

It has been found on numerous occasions that immediately after a prolonged period of sleep deprivation, the first 'recovery' sleep contains unusually large amounts of the EEG slow waves associated with the presumably more restorative stages 3 and 4. Not only is the amount of slow wave sleep increased, but the speed of falling asleep, and the time between sleep onset and first occurrence of stages 3 and 4 is decreased. When the body is very tired it seems to be in a hurry to achieve a lot of slow wave sleep. When Dr W.B. Webb[27] compared the response of young and middle-aged volunteers to two nights of sleep deprivation, he found that older subjects took over twice as long to enter

43

stage 4 after falling asleep (5 minutes for the younger group versus 12 minutes for the older). As both groups then achieved about the same total amount of stage 4, it can be argued that the need for this stage of sleep was equal in both groups, and that sleep in the older person is simply less responsive to the needs created by sleep deprivation. (Although, as pointed out earlier, stage 4 sleep diminishes and, in some individuals, virtually disappears in old age, Dr Webb and his colleagues at the University of Florida have developed a method for 'scoring' stage 4 even when, according to the more traditional criteria described in Chapter 1, it is not there. This is accomplished by ignoring the amplitude or vertical height of the EEG wave, and concentrating only on its frequency. As the EEG slow waves of old age are rather flattened, this modified scoring procedure effectively compensates for the effects of age. Hence the comparison of slow wave sleep in these two age groups.)

Older individuals also appear to respond less efficiently to cumulative occupational sleep loss. In a rather exotic study conducted for the Air Corporations Joint Medical Service, Dr F.S. Preston[28] accompanied the crew of a Boeing 707 on a 15 day transmeridian tour of duty which, after leaving London Heathrow, included flights to Hong-Kong, Tokyo, Honolulu, San Francisco, Singapore, and various other points east before returning to London. Throughout the tour each of the four crew members kept a diary in which they recorded the time and duration of all sleep periods. By converting all diary times to Greenwich Mean Time and then comparing the amount of sleep obtained during each 24 hour period of the tour with the amount of sleep each crew member normally obtained at home, Dr Preston was able to calculate how much sleep each crew member had 'lost' during 15 days of international flying. At the end of the tour it was found that total sleep loss was proportionate to age, with the 51 year-old Captain progressively losing almost 24 hours sleep between the first and fifteenth day away from London, while the 26 year-old Flying Officer began to show a sleep 'debt' only on the thirteenth day. It does appear, then, that with increasing age sleep may adjust less efficiently to the needs of the individual. It is relevant to note that in Dr Ancoli-Israel's[20] study in which the sleep of elderly people was recorded in their own homes, substantial amounts of daytime sleep were recorded within an hour of getting up or going to bed. It is reasonable to suggest that such daytime napping may represent an untimely extension, or a 'spilling-over', of night-time sleep rather than a conceptually discrete sleep event.

While none of the factors considered here (tiredness, boredom, or a fundamental change in the body's ability to regulate the sleep–wakefulness cycle) is independent of daytime sleep, it is extremely unlikely that any one of them is an exclusive cause of napping. Indeed, it is equally unlikely that any one of these factors *could* act independently of the others. Causal influences upon napping are numerous and complex. Nevertheless it does not seem to be the case that daytime sleep among the elderly is wholly a matter of personal choice.

SUMMARY

With increasing age general satisfaction with sleep tends to decline and specific complaints about the continuity, depth, and duration of sleep become more frequent. Laboratory studies using EEG and other measures show age-related changes in the sleep of healthy individuals consistent with these subjective complaints. Advancing age is associated with an increase in the number and the duration of awakenings after sleep onset, a reduction in the total amount of slow wave sleep, and an overall reduction in the total time spent asleep at night. The amount of time spent in bed also shows an age-related increase with some older people apparently trying to compensate for lost sleep by delaying the time at which they get up. In both REM and NREM stages, older people are more vulnerable to disturbance by noise. Older people also seem to adjust less efficiently than younger individuals to disturbances in their sleep routine and from middle age onwards the likelihood of daytime napping increases. Age-related changes in sleep do not appear to affect women and men equally. While women are more likely to report dissatisfaction with their sleep, age-related sleep disturbances, as measured by the EEG, appear to be greater in males. Older men tend to wake more frequently, and according to some reports have a slightly shorter total sleep time than older women. While both sexes show a reduction in the auditory awakening threshold with increased age, the sleep of older women is more likely to be disturbed by noise. A relatively consistent finding from questionnaire studies is that men are more likely to nap during the day. Against this background of apparently normal senescent change in sleeping patterns, age-related events which can affect sleep indirectly will be considered in the next chapter.

NOTES AND REFERENCES

1. The 'sleep system' is conceptual, including all those physiological mechanisms which, under normal circumstances, regulate sleep.
2. S. Smith, Letter to Lady Holland, September 13, 1842. In: *Memoir and Letters of the Reverend Sydney Smith*, Volume II (3rd edition), Longman, Brown, Green, and Longmans, London (1855) pp. 473–4
3. H. Melville, *Moby Dick*, London (1851) p. 29
4. G.G. Sigmond, 'Lectures on Materia Medica and Therapeutics', *Lancet*, 37(1) (1836) pp. 214–20
5. A. McGhie and S.M. Russell, 'The Subjective Assessment of Normal Sleep Patterns', *Journal of Mental Science*, 108 (1962) 642–54
6. I. Karacan, J.I. Thornby, M. Anch, C.E. Holzer, G.J. Warheit, J.J. Schwab, and R.L. Williams, 'The Prevalence of Sleep Disturbance in a Primarily Urban Florida County', *Social Science and Medicine*, 10 (1976) pp. 239–44
7. P. Gerard, K.J. Collins, C. Dore and A.N. Exton-Smith, 'Subjective Characteristics of Sleep in the Elderly', *Age and Ageing,* 7 (supplement) (1978) pp. 55–9
8. K. Gledhill, 'Sleep and the Elderly: Some Psychological Dimensions and their Implications for Treatment' in A. Butler (ed.), *Ageing: Recent Advances and Creative Responses,* Croom Helm, London (1985) pp. 263–77
9. E. Heikkinen, W.E. Waters and Z.J. Brzezinski (eds.), *The Elderly in Eleven Countries: a Sociomedical Survey,* World Health Organization Regional Office for Europe, Copenhagen (1983)
10. R.L. Williams, I. Karacan, and C.J. Hursch, *EEG of Human Sleep: Clinical Applications*, John Wiley and Sons, New York (1974)
11. W.B. Webb, 'Sleep in Older Persons: Sleep Structures in 50- to 60-Year-Old Men and Women', *Journal of Gerontology*, 37 (1982) pp. 581–6
12. I. Feinberg, R.L. Koresko, and N. Heller, 'EEG Sleep Patterns as a Function of Normal and Pathological Aging in Man', *Journal of Psychiatric Research*, 5 (1967) pp. 107–44
13. V. Brezinova, 'The Number and Duration of the Episodes of the Various EEG Stages in Young and Older People', *Electroencephalography and Clinical Neurophysiology*, 39 (1975) pp. 273–8
14. H.P. Roffwarg, J.N. Muzio and W.C. Dement, 'Ontogenetic Development of the Human Sleep-Dream Cycle', *Science*, 152 (1966) pp. 604–19
15. P.N. Prinz, 'Sleep Patterns in the Healthy Aged: Relation-

ship with Intellectual Function', *Journal of Gerontology*, 32 (1977) pp. 179–86

16. H. Zepelin, C.S. McDonald and G.K. Zammit, 'Effects of Age on Auditory Awakening Thresholds', *Journal of Gerontology*, 39 (1984) pp. 294–300

17. J.S. Lukas, 'Noise and Sleep: A Literature Review and a Proposed Criterion for Assessing Effect', *Journal of the Acoustical Society of America*, 58(6) (1975) pp. 1232–42

18. B. Gurland, J. Copeland, J. Kuriansky, M. Kelleher, L. Sharpe and L.L. Dean, *The Mind and Mood of Aging*, Croom Helm, London (1983) See Tables 3–12 (p. 80) and 3–21 (p. 90)

19. W.B. Webb and H. Swinburne, 'An Observational Study of Sleep of the Aged', *Perceptual and Motor Skills*, 32 (1971) pp. 895–8

20. S. Ancoli-Israel, D.F. Kripke, W. Mason and O.J. Kaplan, 'Sleep Apnea and Periodic Movements in an Aging Sample', *Journal of Gerontology*, 40(4) (1985) pp. 419–25

21. For example, Dr E.L. Hartmann suggests that 'Sleep may be connected with restoration after active mental and physical processes; since such processes occur less in old age, less sleep is required', *The Functions of Sleep*, Yale University Press, New Haven and London (1973) p. 83

22. M. Carskadon, J. van den Hoed, and W.C. Dement, 'Sleep and Daytime Sleepiness in the Elderly', *Journal of Geriatric Psychiatry*, 13 (1980) pp. 135–51

23. M.A. Carskadon and W.C. Dement, 'Effects of Total Sleep Loss on Sleep Tendency', *Perceptual and Motor Skills*, 48 (1979) pp. 495–506

24. M.A. Carskadon, E.D. Brown and W.C. Dement, 'Sleep Fragmentation in the Elderly: Relationship to Daytime Sleep Tendency', *Neurobiology of Aging*, 3 (1982) pp. 321–7

25. H. Zepelin, 'A Survey of Age Differences in Sleep Patterns and Dream Recall Among Well-Educated Men and Women', *Sleep Research*, 2 (1973) p. 81

26. Similarities between the sleep of elderly people, and 'circadian desynchronosis' are noted by L.E. Miles and W.C. Dement, 'Sleep and Aging', *Sleep*, 3(2), 119–220, (1980) p. 167

27. W.B. Webb, 'Sleep Stage Responses of Older and Younger Subjects After Sleep Deprivation', *Electroencephalography and Clinical Neurophysiology*, 52 (1981) pp. 368–71

28. F.S. Preston, 'Further Sleep Problems in Airline Pilots on World-Wide Schedules', *Aerospace Medicine*, 44 (1973) pp. 775–82

3

The Indirect Influence of Ageing on Sleep

The age-related structural changes in sleep considered in the previous chapter were described as 'direct' in the sense that they were assumed to result directly from changes in the mechanisms which control sleep and waking. In addition to such directly influenced change, the process of ageing can also affect sleep indirectly as suggested in Figure 2.1. Conceptually indirect influences upon sleep may be divided into those which arise in the internal environment (inside the body), and those which arise in the external environment (outside the body). Both sources of influence will be considered in the present chapter, although each will be approached in a slightly different way. Internal influences are mainly organic or biological in origin and include not only the changes associated with so-called normal ageing, but also those arising from the illnesses and diseases which become more prevalent with increasing age. In the discussion which follows some typical internal changes will be identified and described and their likely influence upon the structure and quality of sleep will be considered.

Events in the external environment, on the other hand, have a less specific and less well documented (though no less real) impact on sleep. Consideration of these influences will focus mainly on the evidence linking some of the major personal, social, and environmental consequences of ageing with disturbed sleep. The overall aim of this chapter is to provide examples rather than an exhaustive list of events and processes which can disrupt sleep in later life. Whether internal or external, organic or personal, many of these events and processes will be superimposed upon existing age-related reductions in the continuity, depth, and duration of sleep. A further aim of the current chapter, then, is to draw attention not only to the variety but also the complexity of events which can underlie disturbed sleep in old age. The emphasis given here to locations inside and outside the body, incidentally, is not meant to infer any philosophical distinction but is merely a convenient although not altogether perfect way of grouping a number of otherwise unrelated events.

AGEING AND DISTURBED SLEEP: INTERNAL EVENTS

Events and processes likely to contribute to disturbed sleep in older individuals are summarised in Table 3.1 and each will be discussed in turn below. First, however, a cautionary note. While many of the influences described in Table 3.1 are 'commonly associated' with disturbed sleep it should not be assumed from this that the events themselves commonly occur. Unlike the fairly widespread changes in sleep described in the previous chapter and defined as 'normal', several of the influences on sleep to be discussed here result from abnormal or pathological ageing processes and may affect only a very small proportion of elderly individuals. Where survey information allows, the extent to which the sleep of the older person is likely to be affected by any of these factors will be considered. [The distinction between normal ageing and abnormal or pathological ageing is used by gerontologists to separate ontogenetic biological changes which inevitably accompany the passage of time from those biological changes which can be attributed to accumulated damage and disease. Whether or not two separate biological ageing processes can be identified and segregated remains a matter for debate.[1] In the present context the distinction is useful if only because, in its absence one must assume either that all age-related changes are benign, which is impractical, or that all age-related change should be regarded as disease, which is silly.]

Changes in bladder function

For a variety of reasons problems associated with voiding urine become more common with increasing age. Changes in the efficiency with which the brain controls the emptying of the

Table 3.1: Age-related factors which can influence sleep indirectly

Biological (internal) factors

Changes in bladder function
Sleep disordered breathing
Limb movements during sleep
Pain and physical discomfort
Iatrogenic causes

Mental health:
  Depression
  Dementia

Social (external) factors

Bereavement
Living alone
Financial hardship
Institutionalisation

bladder, changes in kidney function, changes in the structure of the bladder, or even changes in the circadian rhythmicity of hormones controlling the production of urine can all contribute to symptoms of bladder dysfunction. Many of these problems are more of a nuisance than a major handicap and have little to do with disturbing sleep. However, one of the commonest problems associated with changing bladder function, and one with obvious implications for the continuity of sleep is the need to micturate during the night — nocturia. The generality of this particular complaint was clearly shown in a survey conducted in south London by Professor J.C. Brocklehurst and his colleagues who analysed the responses of 557 individuals aged 65 and over to questions concerning bladder function.[2] In answer to the question 'Do you get up at night to pass urine?' 70 per cent of the men and 61 per cent of the women said that they did. Indeed, about 45 per cent of both the men and women who reported nocturia actually admitted to getting up more than once during the night for this reason. If, then, nocturia is such a prevalent cause of night-time awakenings in the elderly, to what extent does it contribute to the broken sleep which, as we saw in the previous chapter, is so typical of old age? In Dr Irwin

Feinberg's[3] study of the EEG sleep patterns of 15 elderly volunteers described in Chapter 2, he and his colleagues found that while the average number of awakenings per night was 5.4, only one of these awakenings was usually associated with the need to go to the toilet. Among the more physically dependent nursing home patients observed continuously for 36 hours by Webb and Swinburne,[4] a study also described in Chapter 2, 38 per cent of all night-time arousals were attributed to 'bladder control and sundry aches and pains'. Thus, it would appear that nocturia consistently accounts for some but by no means most of the awakenings after sleep onset observed in older people.

Sleep-disordered breathing

Interest in respiratory problems during sleep has increased considerably in recent years with much attention focusing upon the condition of sleep apnoea. While the available research evidence indicates that disordered breathing during sleep becomes more common with increasing age, opinions differ regarding both the medical and personal relevance of this disorder in elderly people. For example, some authorities regard sleep apnoea in the elderly as a terminal illness[5] while others suggest that it may be of little clinical significance in this age group. It is beyond the scope of this book to consider in detail medical controversies which will doubtless be resolved given time and further research. For the present, this section will briefly describe the sleep apnoea syndrome and consider the pertinence of this condition to the quality of sleep *and* quality of life in old age.

   Apnoea (spelled with the dipthong in Britain and without — as apnea — in the United States) means a temporary cessation of breathing. The condition of sleep apnoea, the temporary cessation of breathing during sleep, was first described in 1966 by Dr H. Gastaut and his colleagues working at the French National Institute of Health and Medical Research in Marseilles.[6] Dr Gastaut reported the case of Etienne M, an obese 55 year-old carpenter whose night-time sleep was frequently interrupted by apnoeic periods which could last for up to 40 seconds. Each of these episodes of apnoea was preceded by very loud snoring and terminated by choking gasps, erratic body movements, and a lightening of, or complete awakening from sleep. In this way the unfortunate carpenter never slept for more than 30 minutes at a time, and succeeded in accumulating only about 2 – 3 hours of sleep each night. It is not surprising, therefore, that this man's major complaint was irresistible daytime sleepiness. He regularly fell asleep at work, in his car, or even when talking on the telephone. As at night, each of these periods of daytime sleep was accompanied by stertorous breathing and interrupted by choking gasps.

During the 1970s many of the sleep researchers who had made important contributions to our understanding of normal sleep turned their attention to the identification, diagnosis and treatment of abnormal sleep, and throughout this period centres that specialised in these procedures proliferated in the United States. This increased attention to disorders of sleep allowed for many more cases of sleep apnoea to be examined in detail, and for the diagnostic signs and symptoms of the condition to be refined. In 1976 Dr Christian Guilleminault and his colleagues at the Stanford University School of Medicine published criteria for diagnosing sleep apnoea which are still commonly cited. According to these criteria a sleep apnoea syndrome can be diagnosed if

> During seven hours of nocturnal sleep, at least 30 apneic episodes are observed both in rapid eye movement (REM) and non-rapid eye movement (NREM) sleep, some of which must appear in a repetitive sequence in NREM sleep.[7]

Clinically, sleep apnoeas can be divided into three types: obstructive apnoeas, central apnoeas and mixed apnoeas. Obstructive sleep apnoeas, typified by Dr Gastaut's obese carpenter, appear to result from a gradual relaxation of the throat muscles which, little by little obstructs the airway altogether and prevents the intake of breath. Deprived of oxygen in this way the individual is eventually aroused, the throat muscles return to their pre-sleep state, the airway opens and breathing resumes. When sleep returns, however, the cycle begins again. The loud snoring is probably due to attempts to breathe through a progressively narrowing pharynx, while the gasps and panting after the apnoeic episode indicate that the airway has cleared. Central sleep apnoea, which is not accompanied by noisy or stertorous breathing, appears to result from a disinclination on the part of the central nervous system to initiate breathing. These central apnoeic periods may terminate in a brief arousal from sleep, or in a spontaneous recovery of breathing. A mixed apnoea can mean either a mixture of central and obstructive types in the same apnoeic episode, or a mixture of central and obstructive types occurring separately in the same night's sleep. Sleep apnoea may be associated with headaches, night-time confusion, bed-wetting and, as already described, excessive daytime sleepiness.

When Gastaut and his colleagues published their account of Etienne M little was known about the prevalence of sleep apnoea in the general population. As specialist clinics acquired greater experience in identifying disorders of sleep, it became apparent towards the end of the 1970s that sleep apnoea was extremely common amongst older Americans. For example, in a study reported by Dr Richard Coleman and others[8] it was found that sleep apnoea was the commonest major diagnosis among elderly individuals referred to the Stanford Sleep Disorders Clinic in the two-year period 1978 – 1979. Thus, from a total of 83 referrals, 30 (39 per cent) received this diagnosis. Individuals attending specialist clinics for the assessment of disturbed night-time sleep (or excessive daytime sleepiness) are not, of course, particularly representative of the general population. It might be reasonable to suppose, therefore, that the level of sleep apnoea would be lower than 39 per cent among elderly people at large, and even lower still among groups of elderly individuals who express complete satisfaction with both their sleep and their daytime functioning. Nevertheless, the research evidence suggests that the sleep apnoea syndrome appears to be as common among those Americans who do not complain of sleep–wake problems as it is among those who do. When Dr Mary Carskadon and collaborators[9] at Stanford set out to investigate the relationship between night-time sleep and daytime sleepiness in 24 normal, healthy, uncomplaining elderly volunteers (a study to which reference was made in the previous chapter) they expressed some surprise at finding that nine of their subjects 'qualified' for a diagnosis of sleep apnoea. Even so, the Stanford team found no consistent relationship between disordered breathing and excessive daytime sleepiness in these nine volunteers. The San Diego community study in which the sleep of randomly sampled elderly volunteers was monitored at home shows a similarly high level of sleep apnoea among 'asymptomatic' Americans.

Reporting on this work Dr Sonia Ancoli-Israel and her colleagues estimated that 28 per cent of those living in the 'well-to-do' areas of San Diego show 30 or more apnoeic episodes during sleep.[10]

It would seem, then, that if sleep apnoea is accompanied by complaints of disturbed sleep and by symptoms of excessive daytime sleepiness, then the relationship between the respiratory condition and its daytime consequences is straightforward. If, on the other hand, frequent episodes of sleep apnoea are not accompanied by a complaint then the significance of the apnoea, and the value of diagnosing a sleep apnoea syndrome, are unclear. This lack of clarity has been emphasised by a chorus of doubts recently expressed by sleep researchers. In 1979, commenting on sleep disordered breathing in asymptomatic men, Dr A. Jay Block and others at the University of Florida concluded 'Whether these sleep events have any effect on the longevity or health of these male subjects is not known at present'.[11] In 1980 Dr Carskadon and her team noted 'The possibility that many apneas during sleep may not have a specific deleterious effect in the elderly',[12] and in 1985 Dr Ancoli-Israel suggested that the presence of sleep apnoea as currently defined does 'not always indicate a syndrome of any clinical severity'.[10]

This lack of clarity concerning the significance of sleep apnoea syndrome in uncomplaining elderly people is further emphasised by what might be termed the British experience. In a letter entitled 'Where are the British sleep apnoea patients?'[13] published in the *Lancet* in 1981, a group of sleep researchers and respiratory physicians working at the University of Edinburgh pointed out that while sleep apnoea syndromes appear to be common in the United States, very few cases have been identified in Britain. Indeed, from 120 individuals monitored at the Department of Respiratory Medicine in Edinburgh only two cases of asymptomatic sleep apnoea had been identified. Subsequent research conducted by three of the signatories to the *Lancet* letter (Dr James Catterall, Professor David Flenley and Dr Colin Shapiro) shows that both of these sleep apnoeic individuals, a man of 51 and a woman of 60, were alive and well three years after being identified. Adding their voices to those of American researchers, Dr Catterall and colleagues conclude that, in those over the age of 50 'Sleep disordered breathing may be of little clinical significance'.[14]

As mentioned earlier, sleep apnoea is also associated with body size, so the preponderance of cases in the United States may be related to levels of obesity in that country. Whatever the reason for American–British differences in the incidence of the disorder, many questions relating to the clinical significance of sleep apnoea in old age remain unanswered at the present time. Sleep disordered breathing is clearly an important influence on the continuity of sleep in older people although perhaps, as has been suggested, many older people simply get used to it.

Snoring. As noted above, sleep-disordered breathing and snoring are closely associated. It is not surprising, therefore, that snoring also becomes more common with increasing age. Relationships between ageing and snoring have been thoroughly investigated by Dr E. Lugaresi and his colleagues at the University of Bologna who, over a three year period, collected information on sleeping habits from 5,713 inhabitants of the Republic of San Marino, an independent state situated in north eastern Italy. Results from this massive survey showed that, below the age of 30, only 10 per cent of men and 5 per cent of women admitted to snoring regularly.[15] Between the ages of 60 and 65, however, habitual snorers could be found among 60 per cent of men and 40 per cent of women. Like sleep-disordered breathing, snoring appears to be related to body weight, although the relationship is rather weak. In the San Marino survey 54 per cent of those deemed overweight were habitual snorers, while only 34 per cent of those who were not overweight reported snoring regularly. It could be argued that snoring, as a potential influence upon the continuity of sleep, is more of a problem to one's bed partner than it is to oneself. As men are more likely to snore at any age it might also be argued that this sexually asymmetrical source of disturbed sleep contributes to the finding reported in the previous chapter that women tend to report more dissatisfaction with their sleep than men.

Limb movements during sleep

For reasons that are not at all clear limb movements during sleep become more common with increasing age, in particular jerky movements of the leg. In the sleep disorders clinics of the United States two quite distinct types of leg movement have been described — nocturnal myoclonus (now frequently referred to as Periodic Movements in Sleep or PMS) and the restless leg syndrome. Nocturnal myoclonus (i.e. night-time muscle spasms) describes episodic kicking movements which may (or, like sleep apnoea, may not) disrupt sleep. A similar condition is the curiously named restless leg syndrome in which the sufferer experiences unpleasant pins-and-needles type sensations in the legs which can only be relieved by sometimes quite violent movements. These conditions are not entirely independent and both can be found in the same individual. From recordings made in the homes of sleeping volunteers Dr Ancoli-Israel and her collaborators in San Diego have found that up to 44 per cent of their elderly random sample had 30 or more major leg jerks at night which occurred at a rate of at least 5 jerks per hour.[10] Again, the significance of these events in the absence of any complaint is unclear, at least in so far as the myoclonic or restless individual is concerned. Once again, however, the bed partner may be the more inconvenienced.

Night-time cramps. Again for reasons that are not entirely clear, night-time cramps — painful involuntary contractions of skeletal muscles — are particularly common among elderly people, and are an obvious source of disturbed sleep. It has been suggested that nocturnal cramps in the elderly may be related to daytime exercise levels, salt loss due to diuretic therapy (see below), or to an age-related loss of the nerves which control muscle contractions.[16]

Pain and physical discomfort

Most of us learn at a very early age that sleep can be disturbed by pain. Indirect evidence that older people are more likely to experience pain and physical discomfort is provided by surveys of drug prescribing which have shown on numerous occasions that the use of analgesic drugs (pain-killers) increases steadily with age.[17] This same evidence also shows that these drugs are more likely to be prescribed for women of all ages. Evidence which links pain directly with disturbed sleep in old age is less abundant. Having established *that* many older people are dissatisfied with their sleep relatively few researchers have gone on to ask these people *why* they feel so dissatisfied. Nevertheless, when such questions are asked, the results coincide with commonsense assumptions. In Ken Gledhill's survey of sleep among 109 very elderly people living in Yorkshire, a combination of pain and discomfort was one of the most common reasons offered by those who reported difficulties in sleeping.[18] Specific causes of pain or discomfort in old age are numerous. One source of pain in later life which has quite specific implications for the continuity of sleep, however, is osteoarthritis, a condition in which the smooth articulating surfaces inside a joint degenerate. In the absence of daytime body movements which help to maintain flexibility and reduce pain, arthritic joints tend to become stiff during the night, and sleep is not infrequently disturbed by sudden joint pains when the sufferer moves or attempts to turn over in bed. The extent to which arthritis can disturb sleep is well illustrated by an extensive survey of joint diseases conducted by Drs Acheson and Ginsburg in the city of New Haven, Connecticut, between 1963 and 1967.[19] The two symptoms most commonly associated with arthritis in this survey were joint pains at night and stiffness in the morning. Furthermore it was found that among those with arthritic disabilities, almost one-third of the women and nearly one-quarter of the men complained specifically of difficulty in turning over in bed. Joint pains are extremely prevalent in old age, and in the World Health Organization survey of 'The Elderly in Eleven Countries' mentioned in Chapter 2, joint and back pains were among the most commonly reported of all symptoms.[20]

Iatrogenic causes of sleeplessness

The term 'iatrogenic', once used rather pejoratively by critics of technological medicine has become quite respectable in recent years. Derived from the Greek word *iatros*, meaning physician, iatrogenic describes that group of disorders which are caused by doctors or more accurately, by the treatments doctors provide. Side-effects from prescribed medicines are a common type of iatrogenic disorder. We have already noted that the probability of receiving a prescription for pain-killing drugs increases steadily with age. In fact the use of prescribed medicines generally, and the consequent risk of unwanted side-effects, tends to increase with age in most developed countries. Thus, while the elderly in Britain represent only 15 per cent of the total population, it has been estimated that approximately one-third of the total National Health Service expenditure on medicines is consumed by this age group.[21] This relatively high level of drug usage is not without its risks. In 1980 Professor James Williamson and Dr Joan Chopin of the Department of Geriatric Medicine, University of Edinburgh, reported that over 10 per cent of all geriatric hospital admissions were due wholly or in part to drug side-effects.[22] Different drugs can, of course, produce different side-effects. As regards disturbed sleep in the elderly, at least three types of medicine deserve special attention. They are diuretics (not infrequently referred to as 'water tablets'), some anti-hypertensives (prescribed for the control of high blood pressure) and, paradoxically, hypnotic or sleeping drugs. Diuretics and anti-hypertensives will be considered below while hypnotics will receive detailed attention in Chapters 4 and 5.

Diuretic drugs increase urinary output and are prescribed when the elimination of body fluid is considered beneficial as, for example, in heart failure or in the management of high blood pressure. Diuretics are among the most common of all drugs prescribed for elderly patients. Taken first thing in the morning, the increased urinary output or diuresis produced by these medicines usually reaches a peak during the late morning or early afternoon, and then falls off towards evening. If however the drug is taken much later in the day then the ensuing diuresis will continue until well past bed-time with obvious implications for satisfactory sleep. Elderly people frequently take a variety of different tablets throughout the day. Almost 25 per cent of the hospital admissions studied by Professor Williamson and Dr Chopin were taking 4 to 6 prescribed drugs daily. Under such circumstances, the probability of a diuretic or any other tablet being taken at the wrong time because its effects are not clearly understood, or because instructions have been misunderstood, or because it has been confused for some other tablet are not particularly remote. It is also possible that, once taken, the activity of a diuretic drug may persist longer in older individuals because of age-related reductions in the efficiency with which drugs are metabolised (broken down) and eliminated from the body.

According to some estimates, up to 60 per cent of those over the age of 60 years have hypertension or high blood pressure.[23] Many of these individuals experience no untoward symptoms and learn of their condition only after routine medical examinations. Nevertheless, the evidence shows that even in 'asymptomatic' individuals, untreated hypertension can, after many years, lead to stroke and heart failure. Several different drugs are available for the treatment of this condition including diuretics (which, by reducing the volume of fluid in the blood also reduce blood pressure) and a variety of specific anti-hypertensive agents. Because the aim of drug therapy is to prevent future complications, treatment may commence when the diagnosis is certain and continue throughout the patient's life. While many physicians prefer not to initiate anti-hypertensive therapy in old age unless absolutely necessary, a significant minority of elderly people (over 5 per cent in Williamson and Chopin's study) do receive specific anti-hypertensive medicines. Most of these drugs have been associated with unpleasant side effects and it has frequently been pointed out that, to the patient, the consequences of treatment may seem worse than the condition itself. These side effects frequently include disturbances of sleep. In particular, the drug methyldopa which acts on the central nervous sytem has long been associated with nightmares which, according to one of the most detailed encyclopaedias of side effects 'May occur infrequently'.[24] Disturbances of sleep have also been associated with anti-hypertensive drugs of the beta adrenoceptor blocker type (or 'beta-blockers', so called because they block the stimulating effects of adrenaline on beta receptors), and with the lesser used drug rauwolfia. Like methyldopa, these drugs may also produce nightmares.[25]

Before leaving the topic of drugs, a brief comment on the manner in which sleeping tablets can *disturb* sleep is appropriate. As anyone who has experienced a hangover can testify, drugs can affect the body profoundly not only when they are present, but also when they are withdrawn. Withdrawal effects, sometimes mild, sometimes severe, are particularly noticeable when the drug concerned influences our mood or behaviour directly, as is the case with tranquillisers and their pharmacological relatives, hypnotics (and as is also the case with alcohol). Withdrawal from both tranquillisers and hypnotics is followed by a characteristic sleep disturbance sometimes referred to as 'rebound' insomnia. The extensive use of tranquillisers and hypnotics among elderly people will be discussed in Chapter 4, and the nature of rebound insomnia and its implications are fully described in Chapter 5.

Mental health and sleep

While physical disorders can disrupt sleep in a way that is familiar to most of us, through pain and discomfort, some psychological disorders exert a more subtle influence which can affect not only the continuity, but also the structural characteristics of sleep. Two of the most prevalent psychiatric disorders of old age, depression and dementia, are frequently accompanied by predictable and distressing changes in sleeping patterns. These disorders also contribute to two of the better known stereotypes of old age, with tetchy intolerance suggesting depression, and benign confusion and forgetfulness suggesting dementia. These are popular and powerful images which, for many, touch upon those aspects of ageing which are most feared; dotage and despair. In the discussion which follows, therefore, particular care will be taken to avoid reinforcing negative and inaccurate images of old age. For this reason the prevalence of depression and dementia among the elderly will be considered in some detail.

Depression

The label 'depression' covers a variety of clinically distinct psychological disorders which share the characteristics of melancholic mood, worry, pessimism and lethargy. Depressive mood states also affect sleep and the presence of a subjective sleep complaint is often a diagnostic feature of this distressing condition. The sleep of depressed patients has been examined in numerous laboratory studies over the past 20 years. Summarising the research findings in an article published in the *British Journal of Psychiatry* in 1979 Dr C.-N. Chen[26] concluded that, in general, depressed people 'Have difficulty in falling asleep, frequent shifts of sleep stages, increased time spent awake, early morning awakening, and a considerable reduction in stage 4 sleep'. This description of the sleep of depressed people is, of course, very similar to the description of sleep in healthy elderly people presented in the previous chapter. It does not seem to be the case, however, that most old people are showing signs of incipient depression by sleeping poorly. In a study comparing the psychological profiles of younger (aged 21 – 50) and older (aged 60 and over) dissatisfied sleepers Dr T. Roehrs and colleagues at the Henry Ford Hospital in Detroit concluded that complaints of insomnia are more likely to indicate emotional disturbance in younger persons than they are in older persons.[27] Rather, disruptions of sleep due to age, and those due to mood changes appear to operate independently, as is suggested by the finding that elderly depressives sleep relatively worse than elderly non-depressives. In studies conducted at the University of Pittsburg School of Medicine in the USA, for example, Dr David Kupfer and his colleagues[28] recorded sleep efficiency indexes (i.e. Total Sleep Time divided by Time in Bed; see Table 1.1) of 0.75 and 0.72 for depressed patients aged 41 – 50 and 51 – 60 respectively. For very similar age groups indexes of 0.91 – 0.96 (men and women aged 40 – 49) and 0.92 – 0.93 (men and women aged 50 – 59) were recorded in the Florida studies of physically and psychologically healthy individuals described in the previous chapter. Thus, while older sleepers might sleep poorly, older depressives are likely to sleep *very* poorly. In old age changes in sleep due to depressive illness are superimposed upon, and amplify, those changes attributable to the 'normal' ageing process.

Two changes in sleep, one which is very noticeable and the other covert, appear to be particularly exaggerated in depressed elderly people. The noticeable change concerns early morning awakening, while the less noticeable change concerns a measurement called REM latency, that is the time taken from the onset of sleep until the beginning of the first REM period. Early morning awakening which is unrelated to physical discomfort or pain, but is often associated with a frustrated desire to return to sleep is a common feature of depression and a frequently cited diagnostic symptom. Reductions in REM latency, on the other hand, probably go unnoticed by the depressed person. Nevertheless, it has been suggested by some researchers (notably by Dr David Kupfer whose work is referred to below) that this single EEG index can reliably distinguish the depressed from the non-depressed elderly person. Whatever the precise reason for this biological indicant of mood it does serve to emphasise the intimacy that exists between the architecture of sleep and the emotional state.

The prevalence of depression in the elderly. Detailed community surveys leave little doubt that the social circumstances of old age contribute significantly to the high incidence of depression in this age group. In addition, high levels of physical illness and the ageing of those mechanisms which regulate mood can erode both the motivation and the ability to cope with life's vicissitudes. This interaction between events like bereavement, loneliness, poverty, and personal threat, and the aged individual's coping style makes the placing of depression in the present category of 'Internal' or 'Biological' events as a source of disturbed sleep awkward. It will suffice to acknowledge here that this convenient categorisation of depression does not deny its possible social origins. What, then, is the likelihood of sleep being disturbed by a depressive episode in old age? In the mid-1970s two comprehensive surveys of psychiatric problems among the elderly were conducted simultaneously in New York by Dr Barry Gurland and colleagues and in London by Dr John Copeland and colleagues.[29] Based on detailed information collected from 395 randomly sampled elderly individuals in New York and 445 in London, diagnoses of 'pervasive depression' were applied to 13 per cent of elderly New Yorkers and 12.4 per cent of elderly Londoners. These are 'one-month prevalence rates' which means that, if typical, approximately 12 per cent of the elderly British population will experience a significantly depressed mood in any given month. Assuming an elderly population of 8 million in the UK, this represents 960,000 individuals. The evidence strongly suggests therefore that depression, whether or not it comes to the attention of medical practitioners, is another serious cause of disturbed sleep among the elderly.

Dementia

The conceptual difference between normal and abnormal ageing is perhaps nowhere more emphasised than in the case of dementia. Dementia refers to the intellectual and personal disintegration associated with the abnormal loss of brain cells and is characterised by memory impairments, confusion, and personality changes; with only a few exceptions it is a condition of old age. Clinically, two main types of dementia are recognised, multi-infarct domentia and Alzheimer's disease. In multi-infarct dementia localised areas of brain tissue are repeatedly destroyed when their blood supply is interrupted. As brain cells do not regenerate, the damage resulting from these 'micro-strokes' is necessarily cumulative and is associated with a step-wise behavioural and intellectual decline. Alzheimer's disease, on the other hand, which was first described by the German neurologist Dr Alois Alzheimer[30] in 1907, results from gradual degenerative changes in the structure of the brain, particularly in the neurones or brain cells. In this condition the filaments within the brain cells show characteristically abnormal 'tangles' when seen under the microscope, a feature which distinguishes this from other forms of dementia. On the basis of post-mortem examinations of brain tissue it is now widely accepted that most dementias are of the Alzheimer type, while only the minority result from multiple infarctions. Some dementias combine a mixture of both disorders.

One of the first studies to investigate the sleeping patterns of demented individuals was that conducted by Dr Irwin Feinberg at the State University of New York, and reported in 1967.[3] In addition to measuring the sleep of normal elderly volunteers, as described in the previous chapter, Dr Feinberg also recorded the EEG sleep of 15 inpatients (nine men and six women) diagnosed as having 'chronic brain syndrome' or dementia, and aged between 64 – 92 years. When compared with normal elderly volunteers, demented individuals took longer to get to sleep, awoke more frequently during the night, and stayed awake longer when disturbed. The average total sleep time for these demented patients was 77 minutes less than their non-demented contemporaries, with some of the impaired individuals sleeping for less than three and a half hours per night.

More detailed analyses of changes in sleep due to dementia have since been conducted at the University of Washington by Dr Patricia Prinz and her colleagues.[31] Unlike Feinberg who included several different types of dementia in his 'chronic brain syndrome' group, Dr Prinz and her team were at pains to study only those with so-called senile dementia of the Alzheimer type (or SDAT). The results of these studies show a deterioration not only in the quality of night-time sleep, but also in the distribution of sleep and wakefulness throughout the 24-hour day associated with this form of dementing illness. Compared with normal elderly volunteers, SDAT individuals showed considerably less deep sleep (stages 3 and 4) and REM sleep. They were twice as likely to awaken during the night, and were 20 times as likely to nap during the day. Subsequent research by

Dr Prinz and her team has shown that this overall deterioration in the organisation of sleep is closely related to the degree of behavioural impairment associated with the dementing illness, being least among the mildly demented, and greatest among the moderately and severely demented.[32]

Sleep in dementia thus appears short, shallow, broken and desynchronised. It should be noted however that, in practical terms, the frequent night-time awakening seen in dementing illness represents far more than just a quantitative deterioration in the continuity of sleep. These awakenings are often associated with episodes of apparently aimless wandering. Restless wandering in pursuit of some unclear or forgotten goal is a fairly common feature of dementia which, while problematical at any time of day, can be especially distressing at night. This both applies to the carer, whose sleep is likely to be disturbed, and to the wanderer whose sense of confusion may be increased by darkness or the absence of a usually vigilant supporter. On awakening at night, the elderly demented individual may actively engage in behaviour likely to promote wakefulness which can also exacerbate the existing sleep disturbance. Approaches to this particular problem will be considered in Chapter 6.

The prevalence of dementia. In the early 1960s Dr (now Professor) David Kay of the Royal Victoria Infirmary in Newcastle-upon-Tyne, Dr P. Beamish and Professor Martin Roth conducted a detailed survey of mental disorders among the elderly which has since become something of a research landmark in British geriatric psychiatry.[33] In 1964 these researchers reported that of those people interviewed in Newcastle aged 65 years and over, 4.9 per cent were severely demented and a further 5.2 per cent showed signs of mild dementia. The proportion of severely demented individuals increased steadily with age and was found to be particularly high among those aged over 80. Numerous surveys have since reported very similar age-related trends. In an article published in 1980 Professor Kay and Dr Klaus Bergmann[34] examined the results from 17 different surveys which had been conducted in Europe, the Far East and the United States, and concluded that moderate to severe dementia affects approximately 5 to 8 per cent of those aged over 60, though some estimates vary above and below these figures. [In the US/UK cross-national survey, for example, Dr Gurland and his collaborators found that 4.9 per cent of New Yorkers and only 2.3 per cent of Londoners over the age of 65 were 'pervasively' demented.] In the same article Kay and Bergmann illustrated the age-related increase in levels of dementia by combining the results from three of these surveys. As can be seen from Table 3.2 these studies show a marked rise in the number of demented individuals from just over 2 per cent in the age group 65 – 69 to over 17 per cent among those aged over 80 years.

Table 3.2: Prevalence of organic brain syndromes (dementia) by age and sex

Age	Males (%)	Females (%)	Both sexes (%)
65 – 69	3.9	0.5	2.1
70 – 74	4.1	2.7	3.3
75 – 79	8.0	7.9	8.0
80 +	13.2	20.9	17.7

Source: Kay and Bergmann, 'Epidemiology of Mental Disorders Among The Aged in the Community', in J.E. Birren and R.B. Sloane (eds), *Handbook of Mental Health and Aging* (1980), p. 43, Prentice-Hall, Inc., Engelwood Cliffs, New Jersey (1980). Reprinted with permission.

In order fully to appreciate the significance of these percentages it should be remembered that the elderly population has increased considerably over the past two decades. Consequently, even though prevalence rates might appear to be relatively stable, the *absolute* number of demented individuals has increased. In 1961, for example, close to the time when Kay and his colleagues conducted the Newcastle survey, the British population aged 65 and over numbered 6.1 million. In 1981 it numbered almost 8 million. A 5 per cent prevalence of severe dementia (selected only for the sake of argument) would represent approximately 305,000 individuals in 1961, but would represent approximately 400,000 in 1981 – a rise of almost 100,000 cases of dementia. As the population continues to age demographically, dementia is becoming a major social issue and a growing challenge to both statutory and informal supporters. Professor Kay and Dr Bergmann estimate that between 75 and

80 per cent of all demented individuals are cared for, not in institutions, but 'informally' in the community. Informal care may be provided by a spouse (as women tend to live longer than men, this is especially the case if the demented person is male), or by children, usually female, some of whom may well be over retirement age themselves. It is not unreasonable to conclude, therefore, that while this condition represents an internal influence on the sleep of the demented person, it may also represent an external influence on the sleep of an elderly carer.[35]

AGEING AND DISTURBED SLEEP: EXTERNAL EVENTS

Social and personal changes which in most industrialised nations commonly accompany the process of biological ageing also have implications for the quantity and the continuity of sleep. Retirement, financial limitations, the departure from home of grown-up children, bereavement and the social response to illness represent just some of the events which can, one way or another, affect sleep in later life. However, unlike the biological influences so far considered, the impact of external social events upon sleeping patterns is less specific, less well researched, and is consequently less well documented. Because of this, connections between social change and disturbed sleep are at present based largely upon circumstantial rather than direct 'hard' evidence. Systematic studies comparing the sleep of the elderly poor with that of the elderly affluent, or assessing the impact of loneliness on sleep have yet to be conducted. Nevertheless, it is important not to ignore the possibility that age-related disruptions of sleep do not always result from some immutable biological change but may result instead from some reversible environmental condition. In this section we will consider the implications for sleep of three such environmental conditions associated with ageing: living alone, financial hardship, and institutionalisation.

Living alone

In 1931 only 6.7 per cent of households in Britain consisted of one person living alone.[36] By 1981 this proportion had increased to 21.8 per cent of households,[37] representing about 4.2 million people. Approximately 65 per cent of those now living alone (over 2.8 million) are pensioners. While it cannot be assumed that this personal isolation leads automatically to feelings of loneliness and perhaps despair, the evidence does suggest that for many elderly people, living alone is associated with a number of undesirable emotional consequences. From a survey conducted in 1977 for the British charity Age Concern, Dr Mark Abrams found that elderly people living alone were more likely to report feelings of unhappiness, loneliness, and uselessness.[36] It is relevant to note, therefore, that some researchers have found that extreme fluctuations in mood and morale appear to influence quality of sleep. In a study of psychiatric outpatients reported by Dr Edward Stonehill[38] and others, variations in mood were found to coincide with changes in sleep patterns, extreme sadness being associated with early morning awakening, and anxiety associated with delayed sleep onset.

When living together people also provide each other with a sense of security, reassurance and comfort. When circumstances result in an elderly person living alone, the reassuring presence of others may be replaced by feelings of insecurity which combine with and magnify other adverse social conditions associated with living alone. For example, in the previously mentioned US/UK cross national study of mental health problems in the elderly, Dr Gurland and his colleagues found that in both New York and London those living alone were more likely to be described as 'environmentally disadvantaged'. Disadvantages mentioned in this description included not having a bedroom, finding noise a problem for sleeping, having insufficient heat, and feeling generally unsafe, all of which have implications for quality of sleep.

In addition to the state of being alone, disturbed sleep may also be associated with the cause of being alone. In a comprehensive study of 'Life after a Death'[39] Drs Ann Bowling and Ann Cartwright examined questionnaire responses from 226 elderly widowed females and 124 elderly widowed males approximately 5 – 6 months after their bereavement. When compared with a randomly sampled group of elderly people (only some of whom were widowed), complaints of poor sleep were found to be more than twice as common among the recently bereaved, 50 per cent of whom reported sleeplessness as a problem. Furthermore, 65 per cent of widows and widowers who complained of sleeplessness said that their symptoms had developed, or had become worse, since the death of their spouse. This particular consequence of bereavement is also reflected in the use of sleeping tablets which, as we shall see in the next chapter, are widely prescribed for bereaved women.

Financial hardships

There are doubtless numerous ways in which poverty and hardship can contribute to those physical discomforts which, in old age, can severely affect sleep. It is not unreasonable to speculate, for example, that limited financial resources can lead to an inadequate diet, resulting in feelings of hunger at night, or result in the failure to replace an old and uncomfortable bed. One particular consequence of financial hardship among the elderly with specific implications for sleep quality is the inability of many old people adequately to heat their homes in winter. In Britain one of the first major surveys of winter temperatures in the homes of the elderly was conducted by Dr Ronald Fox and his colleagues during January, February, and March 1972.[40] In all, over 2,000 elderly individuals living in their own homes took part in this study. Although winter temperatures were above average during the period of the survey, the morning temperature in 75 per cent of living rooms was at or below 18.3° centigrade, the minimum temperature recommended for council housing by the Department of the Environment. A further 10 per cent of living rooms were at or below 12° centigrade – very cold indeed.

The impact of such inadequately heated homes on the comfort of elderly occupants is clearly shown in a survey commissioned by the Department of Health and Social Security in Britain, and carried out by Audrey Hunt and others in January and February 1976.[41] The overall purpose of this study was to 'investigate the social circumstances' of people aged over 65 living in the community. Asked if they were warm enough in bed in the winter, 7.6 per cent (194) of the 2558 individuals interviewed said they were not. When asked to provide reasons why they were not warm enough in bed, 39 per cent of these admitted that they could not afford to heat their bedroom. Almost 27 per cent said that they had no means of heating their bedroom, and 9.5 per cent reported having insufficient bedclothes. In Britain today, old age remains a major cause of poverty (where 'poverty' is defined as eligibility for state support from Supplementary Benefits) and poverty remains a major cause of physical discomfort.[42]

Sleeping in institutions

The likelihood of spending even a brief period of time in some form of institutional setting steadily increases with age. Some idea of the probabilities involved can be gleaned from statistics published by the Office of Population Censuses and Surveys (OPCS) in Britain showing the number of persons 'not in private households' at the time of the 1981 national census (the night of 5 – 6 April).[37] The category 'not in private households' includes all those temporarily or permanently resident in hotels, boarding houses, hospitals, nursing homes, and local authority accommodation. Also included in this category are the predominantly younger people resident in defence establishments or detained in Her Majesty's prisons.

Table 3.3: Number of elderly individuals in Britain not in private households on census night 1981

Age-group	Total population	Total and percentage not in households	
25 – 59	23,500,087	425,160	(1.81%)
65 – 69	2,722,492	57,625	(2.12%)
70 – 74	2,318,953	69,070	(2.98%)
75 – 79	1,643,833	85,704	(5.21%)
80 +	1,504,625	218,585	(14.53%)

Source: OPCS[37]

As can be seen from Table 3.3 the likelihood of not being in a private household increases steadily throughout old age. Estimates suggest that at any one time almost half a million elderly people in Britain are in some form of institutional care, which includes 131,000 in local authority residential homes, 70,000 in private and voluntary homes, and 31,000 in voluntary hospitals and private nursing homes.[43] A further 220,000 elderly individuals occupy National Health Service hospital beds.[44] That the benefits of hospital or residential care are sometimes gained at the cost of disturbed sleep is strongly suggested by trends in the use of sleeping tablets. Prevalence rates of sleeping drug usage among the elderly are 2 – 3 times higher in institutions than they are in the community. This topic will receive detailed attention in Chapter 4. However, a brief glance at Tables 4.2 and 4.3 shows that while prevalence rates of hypnotic usage among the elderly in the community range from 6 – 33 per cent, those from hospitals, residential homes, and nursing homes range from 22 to over 50 per cent. Among hospital inpatients where sleeplessness may be related to the cause of admission, this is not altogether unexpected. However, it is difficult to employ the same argument for residential homes where, in many cases, residents are frail rather than ill. In addition to the physical discomforts of ill health, then, the institutional environment itself may degrade sleep quality perhaps because of its initial strangeness, its psychological impact, or because of its sheer disregard for peace and quiet!

Studies conducted both in Britain and in North America show that excessive noise is an all too common cause of irritation, stress, and sleeplessness in hospitals. As noted in the previous chapter, auditory awakening thresholds (i.e. the minimum amount of noise required to wake a sleeping person) tend to decrease with increasing age making the problem of noisy hospitals particularly relevant among the elderly. In a study conducted by B. Ann Hilton[45] in Canada sound levels were monitored in the vicinity of selected hospital patients. It was found that in some specialised units, sound levels remained equivalent to that produced by heavy traffic throughout a 24 hour period. Even in those wards where sound levels fell at night, intermittent noises in excess of 50 decibels (equivalent to a passing car) were frequently recorded. (The US Environmental Protection Agency actually recommends a sound level of 35 decibels for hospitals at night.) In a report published in the *British Medical Journal* in 1986, Richard Soutar and Dr John Wilson[46] describe similar night-time sound levels in general medical wards at Ninewells Hospital in Dundee, Scotland. In both studies noise was identified by patients as a major cause of disturbed sleep. Soutar and Wilson, for example, report that 28 out of 91 patients interviewed claimed that their sleep was worse in hospital. Of the 28 disturbed sleepers, nine attributed this disturbance to noise. Of course, sound does not have to be. perceived as noise in order to antagonise sleep. Some sounds are by their nature emotionally disturbing, for example dripping or bubbling. And for some the mere presence of a sound, like the gentle snoring of a sleeping neighbour in a shared room, is enough to generate an emotional state incompatible with sleep.

SUMMARY

In addition to the senescent changes which directly influence the structure and quality of sleep, advancing age is also associated with an increasing number of events and processes which can influence and disturb sleeping patterns indirectly. These indirect influences upon sleep can arise in the internal (biological) or in the external (social) environments, and can include the consequences of so-called normal ageing as well as age-related pathological or disease processes. The present chapter has focused upon some of the more common organic and social events which are known to affect sleep, or which might reasonably be expected to affect sleep in old age. Relative to younger adults elderly people are more likely to experience joint pains and physical discomforts at night, to breathe irregularly, snore, and emit jerky leg movements during sleep, to take medicines which interfere with their sleep, and have their sleep disturbed by the need to micturate. Characteristic patterns of sleep disturbance are also associated with the two most common psychiatric disorders of old age — depression and dementia. The social consequences of ageing also have implications for sleep quality. Old age contributes to the likelihood of living alone, experiencing financial hardship, and spending at least some time in an institution, all of which can and frequently do result in disturbed sleep.

NOTES AND REFERENCES

1. A discussion of these issues can be found in D.B. Bromley, *The Psychology of Human Ageing*, 2nd Edition, Penguin, Harmondsworth (1975) pp. 114–18

2. J.C. Brocklehurst, J. Fry, L.L. Griffiths and G. Kalton, 'Dysuria in Old Age', *Journal of the American Geriatrics Society*, 19 (1971) pp. 582–92
3. I. Feinberg, R.L. Koresko and N. Heller, 'EEG Sleep Patterns as a Function of Normal and Pathological Aging in Man', *Journal of Psychiatric Research*, 5 (1967) pp. 107–44
4. W.B. Webb and H. Swinburne, 'An Observational Study of Sleep of the Aged', *Perceptual and Motor Skills*, 32 (1971) pp. 895–8
5. L.E. Miles and W.C. Dement, 'Sleep and Aging', *Sleep*, 3(2) 119–220 (1980), p. 184. These reviewers conclude that 'Most sleep disorders clinicians view upper airway sleep apnea as a terminal illness'
6. H. Gastaut, C.A. Tassinari and B. Duron, 'Polygraphic Study of the Episodic Diurnal and Nocturnal (Hypnic and Respiratory) Manifestations of the Pickwick Syndrome', *Brain Research*, 2 (1966) pp. 167–86
7. C. Guilleminault, A. Tilkian and W.C. Dement, 'The Sleep Apnea Syndromes', *Annual Review of Medicine*, 27 (1976) pp. 465–84
8. R.M. Coleman, L.E. Miles, C. Guilleminault, V.P. Zarcone, J van den Hoed and W.C. Dement, 'Sleep-Wake Disorders in the Elderly: A Polysomnographic Analysis', *Journal of the American Geriatrics Society*, 19 (1981) pp. 289–96
9. M.A. Carskadon, E.D. Brown and W.C. Dement, 'Sleep Fragmentation in the Elderly: Relationship to Daytime Sleep Tendency', *Neurobiology of Aging*, 3 (1982) pp. 321–7
10. S. Ancoli-Israel, D.F. Kripke, W. Mason and O.J. Kaplan, 'Sleep Apnea and Periodic Movements in an Aging Sample', *Journal of Gerontology*, 40 (1985) pp. 419–25
11. A.J. Block, P.G. Boysen, J.W. Wynne and L.A. Hunt, 'Sleep Apnea, Hypopnea, and Oxygen Desaturation in Normal Subjects', *New England Journal of Medicine*, 300 (1979) pp. 513–17
12. M.A. Carskadon, J. van den Hoed and W.C. Dement, 'Sleep and Daytime Sleepiness in the Elderly', *Journal of Geriatric Psychiatry*, 13 (1980) pp. 135–51
13. C.M. Shapiro, J.R. Catterall, I. Oswald and D.C. Flenley, 'Where Are All The British Sleep Apnoea Patients?', *Lancet*, ii (1981) p. 523
14. J.R. Catterall, P.M.A. Calverly, C.M. Shapiro, D.C. Flenley and N.J. Douglas, 'Breathing and Oxygenation during Sleep Are Similar in Normal Men and Normal Women', *American Review of Respiratory Diseases*, 132 (1985) pp. 86–8
15. E. Lugaresi, F. Cirignotta, G. Coccagna and C. Piana, 'Some Epidemiological Data on Snoring and Cardiocirculatory Disturbance', *Sleep*, 3 (1980) pp. 221–4
16. See R.W. Warne, 'Cramps, Stiffness and Restless Legs', *Current Therapeutics*, October (1984) pp. 35–9
17. See, for example, D.C.G. Skegg, R. Doll and J. Perry, 'Use of Medicines in General Practice', *British Medical Journal*, 1 (1977) pp. 1561–3
18. K. Gledhill, 'Sleep and The Elderly: Some Psychological Dimensions and their Implications for Treatment', in A. Butler (ed.)

Ageing: Recent Advances and Creative Responses, Croom Helm, London (1985) pp. 263–77

19. R.M. Acheson and G.N. Ginsburg, 'New Haven Survey of Joint Diseases XVI. Impairment, Disability, and Arthritis', *British Journal of Preventive and Social Medicine*, 27 (1973) pp. 168–76

20. E. Heikkinen, W.E. Waters and Z.J. Brzezinski, *The Elderly in Eleven Countries. A Sociomedical Survey*, World Health Organization Regional Office for Europe, Copenhagen (1983) p. 40 and Table 25

21. After J. Crooks, A.H.M. Shepherd and I.H. Stevenson, 'Drugs and the Elderly: The Nature of the Problem', *Health Bulletin*, 33 (1975) pp. 222–7

22. J. Williamson and J.M. Chopin, 'Adverse Reactions To Prescribed Drugs in the Elderly: A Multicentre Investigation', *Age and Ageing*, 9(2) (1980) pp. 73–80

23. Not all clinicians agree on what constitutes hypertension in old age. The estimates reported here are for a systolic pressure of 160 mm Hg or more and/or a diastolic pressure of 95 mm Hg or more. After B.O. Williams, 'The Cardiovascular System' in M.S.J. Pathy (ed.), *Principles and Practice of Geriatric Medicine*, John Wiley and Sons Ltd., Chichester, (1985) p. 478

24. J.A. Steiner 'Antihypertensive Drugs' in M.N.G. Dukes (ed.), *Meyler's Side Effects of Drugs*, 10th Edition, Elsevier, Amsterdam (1984) p. 358

25. See, for example H.J. Waal, 'Propranalol Induced Depression', *British Medical Journal*, 2 (1967), p. 50

26. Char-Nie Chen, 'Sleep, Depression and Antidepressants', *British Journal of Psychiatry*, 135 (1979) pp. 385–402

27. T. Roehrs, W. Lineback, F. Zorick and T. Roth, 'Relationship of Psychopathology to Insomnia in the Elderly', *Journal of the American Geriatrics Society*, 30 (1982) pp. 312–15

28. D.J. Kupfer, C.F. Reynolds, R.F. Ulrich, D.H. Shaw and P.A. Coble, 'EEG Sleep, Depression and Aging', *Neurobiology of Aging*, 3 (1982) pp. 351–60

29. B. Gurland, J. Copeland, J. Kuriansky, M. Kelleher, L. Sharpe and L.L. Dean, *The Mind and Mood of Ageing*, Croom Helm, London (1983)

30. A. Alzheimer, 'Uber Eine Eigenartige Erkrankung der Hirnrinde' (On a peculiar disease of the cerebral cortex) Allg. Z. Psychiat. Translation: R.H. Wilkins and I.A. Brody, 'Alzheimer's Disease', *Archives of Neurology*, 21 (1969) pp. 109–10

31. P.N. Prinz, E.R. Peskind, P.P. Vitaliano, M.A. Raskind, C. Eisdorfer, N. Zemcuznikov and C.J. Gerber, 'Changes in the Sleep and Waking EEGs of Nondemented and Demented Elderly Subjects', *Journal of the American Geriatrics Society*, 30 (1982) pp. 86–93

32. P.N. Prinz, P.P. Vitaliano, M.V. Vitiello, J. Bokan, M. Raskind, E. Peskind and C. Gerber, 'Sleep, EEG and Mental Function Changes in Senile Dementia of the Alzheimer's Type', *Neurobiology of Aging*, 3 (1982) pp. 361–70

33. D.W.K. Kay, P. Beamish and M. Roth, 'Old Age Mental Disorders in Newcastle upon Tyne. Part 1: A Study of Prevalence',

British Journal of Psychiatry, 110 (1964) pp. 146–58

34. D.W.K. Kay and K. Bergmann, 'Epidemiology of Mental Disorders Among the Aged in the Community' in J.E. Birren and R.B. Sloane (eds.) *Handbook of Mental Health and Aging*, Prentice-Hall, Engelwood Cliffs (1980) pp. 34–56

35. In studies of the problems faced by those caring for demented relatives at home, Gilleard found night-time wandering to be one of the major problems reported by caregivers. See C.J. Gilleard, *Living With Dementia. Community Care of the Elderly Mentally Infirm*, Croom Helm, London, (1984) Table 5.1, p. 69

36. The figures for 1931 are summarised in M. Abrams, *Beyond Three Score and Ten: a First Report on a Survey of the Elderly*, Age Concern England, Mitcham, (1978) p. 10

37. Office of Population Censuses and Surveys, *Census (1981) Great Britain Summary*, HMSO, London, Table D (1983)

38. E. Stonehill, A.H. Crisp and J. Koval, 'The Relationship of Reported Sleep Characteristics to Psychiatric Diagnosis and Mood', *British Journal of Medical Psychology*, 49 (1976) pp. 381–91

39. A. Bowling and A. Cartwright, *Life After A Death. A Study of the Elderly Widowed*, Tavistock Publications, London. See Table 34 (1982) p. 97

40. R.H. Fox, P.M. Woodward, A.N. Exton-Smith, D.V. Donnison and M.H. Wicks, 'Body Temperatures in the Elderly. A National Study of Physiological, Social and Environmental Conditions', *British Medical Journal*, 1 (1973) pp. 200–6

41. A. Hunt, *The Elderly at Home*, HMSO, London. See Table 10.10.2 (1978) p. 80

42. For a brief, though detailed discussion of the relationship between poverty and old age see D. Jordan, 'Poverty and the Elderly' in V. Carver and P. Liddiard (eds) *An Ageing Population*, Hodder and Stoughton, Sevenoaks (1978)

43. Department of Health and Social Security, *Growing Older*, HMSO, London (1980)

44. N.W. Chaplin, (ed.) *The Hospitals and Health Services Yearbook*, Institute of Health Service Administrators, London (1981)

45. B.A. Hilton 'Noise in Acute Patient Care Areas', *Research in Nursing and Health*, 8 (1985) 283–91

46. R.L. Soutar and J.A. Wilson, 'Does Hospital Noise Disturb Patients?', *British Medical Journal*, 292 (1986) p. 305

4

Hypnotic Drugs and their Use Among Elderly People

Between February and July 1981 some 12,000 households across Canada took part in one of the largest surveys of physical activity patterns ever undertaken – the Canada Fitness Survey. During the course of this immense study over 22,000 Canadians, ranging in age from 10 to 97 years, completed an 11 page questionnaire. They answered questions about their participation in recreational and sporting activities, and their attitudes toward physical fitness and health. In one of the questions participants were asked to choose from a list of 'health related activities' those which they considered important for achieving a sense of personal wellbeing. These activities, and the importance attached to each are shown in Figure 4.1. As can be seen, not only was 'getting enough rest and sleep' the most highly rated among them, but it was *equally* highly rated by all age groups.[1]

Unfortunately, while the importance attached to sleep does not appear to change with increasing age, actual quality of sleep certainly does. As we have seen in the previous two chapters sleep becomes shorter, lighter, more broken, more vulnerable to disruption, and less satisfying as we get older. Given the consistently high value placed upon rest and sleep throughout life, it is not particularly surprising, then, that the use of sleeping drugs increases steadily with age. The pattern of sleeping drug usage shown in Figure 4.2, for example, is typical for most developed countries. Usage rises throughout early and late adulthood, increases sharply in middle age, and continues to increase steadily until well into the eighth decade.[2]

At first sight, the use of sleeping tablets may appear to be a reasonable and appropriate response to age-related reductions

75

Figure 4.1: Percentage of people in three age groups reporting that certain behaviours are important for achieving personal wellbeing; results from a survey of approximately 22,000 people living in Canada

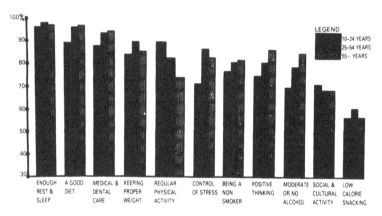

Source: *Fitness and Aging*, Canada Fitness Survey, 506–294 Albert Street, Ottawa, K1P 6E6, Canada, (1982).

Figure 4.2: Age and consumption of sleeping drugs

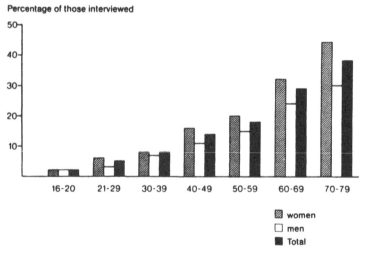

Note: Data from a representative investigation carried out in West Germany. The respondents were asked if they 'sometimes' took sleep medication.
Source: R. Spiegel and A. Azcona 'Sleep and Its Disorders' in M.S.J. Pathy (ed.) *Principles and Practice of Geriatric Medicine,* John Wiley and Sons Ltd, Chichester, (1985). Reprinted with permission.

in sleep quality; after all, these tablets are prescribed by doctors who have our best interests at heart. There are, however, risks as well as benefits associated with the use of all drugs, and hypnotics are no exception. In this and the following chapter I will focus upon the role of hypnotic drugs in the treatment of sleep problems in old age and, in particular, consider both the effects and side-effects of these widely used medicines. This temporary shift in emphasis away from sleep *per se* introduces both a new subject and a new vocabulary. Assuming no prior knowledge on the part of the reader, I will develop this discussion of hypnotics by first addressing three basic questions: first, 'What are hypnotic drugs?'; second, 'What effects do hypnotic drugs have on sleep?'; and third, 'To what extent are hypnotic drugs used among elderly people?'

WHAT ARE HYPNOTIC DRUGS?

The word 'hypnotic' stems from the Greek *hypnos* meaning sleep. In Greek mythology a minor deity of the same name — Hypnos — flitted between Hades and the living world exerting his soporific influence on mortals and immortals alike. In clinical pharmacology a drug is described as a hypnotic if it promotes sleep. (Used in this context, the term 'hypnotic' should not be confused with the trance-like state popularised in the late eighteenth century by Friedrich Anton Mesmer. The hypnotic trance, so-called because of its supposed similarity to sleep-walking, is in fact misnamed since hypnosis is not a state of sleep).[3] In addition to promoting sleep, hypnotic drugs have another important and frequently overlooked property: they reduce anxiety. Hypnotics and tranquillisers are the same in virtually everything but name.[4] The major differences between them are semantic rather than pharmacological. If, for example, a certain drug is taken during the daytime to alter mood and to control anxiety, it will probably be called a tranquilliser. If the same drug is taken only in a single dose at night to promote sleep, it will probably be called a hypnotic. Hypnotics and tranquillisers not only share the same therapeutic effects but, as we shall see later, they also create the same problems.

There is nothing new about the use of sleeping drugs. The medicinal value of naturally occurring substances which can relieve pain and sleeplessness has long been recognised in human societies, and the poppy *Papaver somniferum* has, for at least the past two thousand years, provided a rich source of pain-killing and sleep-inducing preparations. From this single plant comes opium, heroin, morphine, laudanum, and other 'opiates', each of which can induce sleep if taken in sufficient quantities. Unfortunately these drugs also interfere with other essential functions like breathing or the reflex mechanism which makes us cough. As an alternative to such naturally occurring substances, research chemists and pharmacologists turned their attention to the manufacture or 'synthesis' of compounds that were safe to use and specific in their action, affecting sleep and little else. One of the first 'true' hypnotic drugs, chloral hydrate, was first synthesised in 1832 and introduced towards the end of the nineteenth century.[5] Chloral derivatives (for example the tablet dichloralphenazone) continue to be used today. In 1903 the first barbiturate drugs were introduced which, throughout the first half of the twentieth century, became the most widely used of all hypnotics. However, as mentioned in Chapter 1, barbiturates suffered from at least two major drawbacks, they were often fatal in overdose and they became widely abused. Because of these disadvantages, barbiturates fell from favour and, at least in Europe, are now rarely used in the treatment of problem sleep.

Most of the hypnotics and tranquillisers currently prescribed belong to the pharmacological 'family' of drugs called benzodiazepines. Introduced in the early 1960s, benzodiazepines soon replaced the more toxic and more habit-forming barbiturates as the drugs of choice for treating both anxiety and sleeplessness. The first of these new tranquillisers, chlordiazepoxide, was developed by Roche Laboratories in Europe and was first introduced into the United States under the trade name 'Librium' in 1960. Soon to follow were diazepam ('Valium') in 1963 and nitrazepam ('Mogadon'), the archetypal benzodiazepine hypnotic, in 1965.[6] [For those unfamiliar with esoteric pharmaceutical conventions it should be pointed out that most drugs have at least two names, a non-proprietary or generic name and a proprietary or trade name. The non-proprietary name is that under which the drug is registered and remains the same no matter who manufactures it. Proprietary or trade names, on the other hand, are the imaginative and eye-catching titles that drug companies give to their products when they are marketed. While a drug may have one generic name, it can have a variety of trade names. In Britain, for example, the drug known generically as nitrazepam is marketed by six different companies as 'Somnite', 'Mogadon', 'Nitrados', 'Remnos', 'Surem', and 'Unisomnia' respectively. Generic names will be used preferentially here. The generic names of benzodiazepines, incidentally, frequently end in 'pam' or 'am'].

What effects do hypnotics have on sleep?

Unlike those drugs developed in the late nineteenth or early twentieth century, benzodiazepines were introduced at a time when sleep, and the impact of drugs upon sleep, could be accurately and precisely measured. As a result there now exists a detailed sleep laboratory profile for most of the hypnotic products currently prescribed. The procedure most usually employed to assess the effects of a new hypnotic drug is the 'clinical trial', during which the sleep of volunteers is recorded before, during and after a course of sleeping tablets. In addition to attending the EEG laboratory at intervals throughout the trial, these volunteers may also be asked to evaluate their own sleep by completing questionnaires or visual analogue scales, as described in Chapter 1. In laboratory studies as in life, people are frequently influenced by their own expectations. Volunteers taking part in a clinical trial might, for example, rate their sleep as improved simply because they expect it to improve. Or they might actually sleep better not because the tablets are pharma-cologically effective, but because the presence of the researcher, and the laboratory environment are so reassuring.

Researchers, on the other hand, can quite unintentionally distort laboratory results in line with their expectations. For instance, they may unwittingly 'cue' certain positive responses from volunteers by saying things like, 'Well now, don't you think you had a much better sleep last night?' In either case, both the observer and the observed can introduce bias into research findings. To minimise this bias clinical trials employ what is called a 'double blind' technique, which means that in addition to the real or 'active' hypnotics the volunteer also takes inert dummy tablets which look like, and should taste and smell like, the active drug. Active and dummy hypnotics are then administered in a sequence known only to a third person, leaving both the volunteer and the researcher 'blind' to the nature of each tablet. On completion of the trial the researcher learns when active and dummy drugs were taken, and divides the EEG sleep recordings and behavioural ratings accordingly. By convention the dummy drug is referred to as a 'placebo', the Latin for 'I will please'. (The use of this particular term derives from the time-honoured medical practice of placating troublesome patients by giving them some inactive physic, a placebo, with the assurance that it will do them some good. Often it did.)

In general hypnotic drugs reduce sleep onset latency, decrease the amount of wakefulness intervening during sleep, and consequently increase total sleep time. Figure 4.3, for example, shows the results from a double-blind trial of the benzodiazepine loprazolam which was taken in a 1 mg dose each night for a period of three weeks.[7] Placebos were taken for one week before this period (the 'baseline' week), and for one week afterwards (the 'withdrawal' week). Relative to the baseline week, which can be considered as the norm for these volunteers, the three drug weeks show a marked reduction in total intervening wakefulness. (There are other equally important aspects of this figure to which we shall return in due

Figure 4.3: The effect of an intermediate half-life hypnotic (Loprazolam) on intervening wakefulness

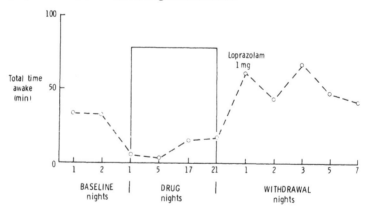

TOTAL MINUTES OF WAKEFULNESS ACCUMULATED
AFTER THE FIRST ONSET OF SLEEP
(Each point is the average for 9 middle-aged volunteers)

Note: Placebo (dummy) tablets were taken during the 'baseline' and 'withdrawal' periods.
Source: Adam *et al.* (1984).[7] Reprinted with permission.

Figure 4.4: The effect of an intermediate half-life hypnotic (Loprazolam 1 mg) on subjective ratings of sleep quality

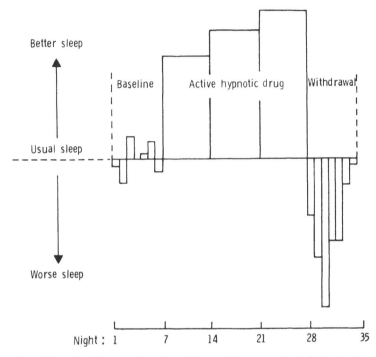

RATINGS OF SLEEP QUALITY BEFORE, DURING AND AFTER
3 WEEKS OF HYPNOTIC DRUG USAGE

Note: Visual-analogue ratings (see Chapter 1) were made daily by twelve middle-aged volunteers; placebo tablets were taken during the 'baseline' and 'withdrawal' periods.

course.) Hypnotic drugs also affect the way we feel about our sleep. Figure 4.4 shows the influence of the same drug, loprazolam, on daily visual analogue ratings of sleep quality.[8] Again, the baseline week can be considered as the norm for these volunteers. Satisfaction with sleep shows a dramatic improvement after the first dose of active hypnotic, and is maintained at an elevated level until the drug is withdrawn. The effects of drug withdrawal, by the way, will be considered in the next chapter. In passing, however, we may note that when a regularly taken hypnotic is discontinued the original drug effects can be reversed, with both intervening wakefulness and

81

dissatisfaction with sleep increasing relative to their original baseline levels.

It has frequently been pointed out that drug-induced sleep does not resemble 'natural' sleep. In addition to the effects already mentioned most drugs of the benzodiazepine type reduce total REM and slow wave sleep, and produce a reciprocal increase in stage 2. The precise significance of these changes is not clear, although they appear to be relatively harmless events. In an article sensibly entitled 'Are Poor Sleepers Changed Into Good Sleepers by Hypnotic Drugs?'[9] Dr Kirstine Adam of the University of Edinburgh points out that while hypnotics decrease total slow wave sleep as recorded by the EEG, some of the biological processes associated with this sleep stage continue unabated, and she concludes that 'It may be that these drugs merely interfere with the generation of electrical brain waves without disturbing the biological processes associated with sleep'.

While hypnotics improve sleep quality in the short term, they do not continue to be effective if taken continuously over long periods of time. Regular usage produces 'tolerance' whereby the body becomes accustomed to the drug, larger doses of which are then required in order to achieve the original effect. Look again at Figure 4.3. Throughout the 3 weeks of drug usage intervening wakefulness creeps back towards its original level as the drug becomes less effective. In 1980 the Committee on the Review of Medicines (a body set up under the Medicines Act of 1968 to assess the safety, quality, and efficacy of drugs marketed in the United Kingdom) concluded that 'Most hypnotics tend to lose their sleep-promoting properties within three to 14 days [of usage]'.[10] This conclusion may underestimate the effective 'lifespan' of some hypnotics. In an article published in the *British Medical Journal* in 1982, for example, Professor Ian Oswald and others reported that both nitrazepam and lormetazepam can sustain an improvement in subjectively rated sleep quality for up to 32 weeks.[11] Nevertheless, as is clear from Figure 4.3, some of the effects of hypnotics on the EEG structure of sleep begin to wane within the first two weeks of usage. All hypnotics become less effective with regular use.

So far we have considered only the similarities among hypnotic drugs, and paid little attention to their differences. Not all hypnotics are the same, and one characteristic on which they may differ considerably is the length of time for which they

Table 4.1: Plasma half-lives of some typical benzodiazepine sedative–hypnotic drugs

Non-proprietary name	Half-life (hours) of drug or active metabolites
Long half-life	
Diazepam	100
Flurazepam	50 – 100
Nitrazepam*	20 – 40
Intermediate half-life	
Lorazepam	12
Temazepam	10 – 17
Oxazepam	12
Lormetazepam*	13 – 14
Loprazolam*	15
Short half-life	
Triazolam	3

Note: * not available in the USA.
Sources: Lader (1983);[34] Hugget *et al.* (1981);[35] Humpel *et al.* (1979);[36] Humpel *et al.* (1980);[37] Jochemsen *et al.* (1983);[38] Jochemsen *et al.* (1983)[39]

remain active. Like radioactivity, a drug's duration of action is usually described in terms of its half-life, that is, the time required for peak drug concentrations in the body to be reduced by half (see Table 4.1). The drug loprazolam, for example, has a half-life of about 15 hours, while for nitrazepam the half-life can exceed 30 hours. Consequently the sedative effects of nitrazepam are likely to persist for longer than those of the shorter-acting loprazolam. Drug concentrations are reduced by the process of metabolism which breaks the drug down into more easily excreted 'metabolites'. Some of these metabolites are themselves active hypnotics which may remain active for longer than the parent compound. Both diazepam and flurazepam, for example, release the active metabolite N-desmethyldiazepam, a drug with sedative properties which has a half-life of about 100 hours. The half-lives of some typical benzodiazepine hypnotics are shown in Table 4.1. While some drugs are inherently shorter acting than others, the speed with which the drug is eliminated from the system frequently depends upon the age of that system. In general, older bodies are less efficient than younger bodies at eliminating drugs, a point to which we shall also return in Chapter 5. Benzodiazepines can also differ in terms of their potency, with a small dose of one drug being equivalent to a relatively larger dose of another drug (larger, that is, in terms of its mg weight). For example 1 mg of lormetazepam possesses roughly the same sleep inducing properties as 5 mg of nitrazepam; thus lormetazepam is the more potent drug.

Hypnotic drug usage among the elderly

As the variety of available mood altering and hypnotic drugs increased throughout the 1950s and 1960s, so too did socio-logical interest in the prescribing and use of these medicines. [Drugs which alter mood or behaviour, including tranquillisers, hypnotics, and anti-depressants, are known collectively as 'psychotropic' drugs. While clearly jargon, the term is at least economical and will be used here.] From detailed surveys of psychotropic drug usage it soon became clear that, irrespective of where these surveys were conducted the findings were remarkably consistent. Reports from the United Kingdom, the United States, Canada, Sweden and elsewhere all consistently showed that the use of psychotropic drugs increased with age. Closer analysis showed that hypnotic drugs were principally responsible for producing this age-related trend. More so than for any other psychotropic, the use of hypnotic drugs increased steadily with advancing age. It is for this reason that the trend shown in Figure 4.2 can be considered as typical.

Age-related trends tell us little about the absolute prevalence of drug usage. In other words, older people may take more hypnotics than younger people, but what proportion of older people *do* take hypnotics? Tables 4.2 and 4.3 summarise the findings of 23 different surveys of drug use conducted in both Britain and the United States, and reported between 1962 and 1984.[12] Collectively, these survey findings show that since the early 1960s elderly people have remained the most popular 'target' group for hypnotic drugs. Two other important character-

Table 4.2: Studies reporting rates of hypnotic drug usage among the elderly living at home

Study: Authors (date reported)	Origin	Age of Sample	Prevalence rates (%) Men	Women	Total
McGhie and Russell (1962)	UK	75+	25.0	45.0	–
Manheimer et al. (1968)	USA	60+	10.0	13.0	11.2
Mellinger et al. (1971)	USA	60+	9.0	13.0	11.5
Stevenson and Gaskell (1971)	UK	70+	–	–	14.6
Dunnell and Cartwright (1972)	UK	65+	–	–	18.1
Parry et al. (1973)	USA	60+	7.0	8.0	7.6
Gruer (1975)	UK	65+	–	–	19.0
Wilks (1975	UK	65+	6.4	5.5	5.9
Law and Chalmers (1976)	UK	75+	–	–	8.6
Karacan et al. (1976)	USA	70+	12.3	22.0	18.3
Skegg et al. (1977)	UK	75+	21.4	29.9	27.3
Gerard et al. (1978)	UK	65+	18.0	40.0	33.0
Williamson and Chopin (1980)	UK	–	22.6	22.0	22.2
Murray et al. (1981)	UK	65+	6.1	12.0	9.7
Stewart et al. (1982)	USA	65+	5.4	7.2	6.6

– Information not reported.
Source: Morgan (1983)[12]

istics of usage are also clear: first, hypnotic drug use tends to be higher among elderly people in institutions than among elderly people living at home. And second, usage tends to be higher among women than among men. We will consider these two points in turn.

The prevalence rates shown in Table 4.2 suggest that, on average, about 10 to 15 per cent of the elderly population living at home consume prescribed hypnotic drugs. From a methodological point of view the exact figure frequently depends upon how 'elderly' is defined. If, for example, the prevalence rates shown in Table 4.2 are averaged according to the minimum age of the sample, then the overall average prevalence rate for the 60+ age groups is much lower than the average prevalence for the 75+ age groups. (This probably explains why usage among elderly Americans appears, from Table 4.2, to be less than that among elderly Britons. The American samples tend to be younger.) Table 4.3, on the other hand, shows that hypnotic drug usage among the elderly in various types of institution averages about 35 per cent, over twice that of the community

Table 4.3: Studies reporting prevalence rates of hypnotic drug usage among elderly people in institutions

Study: Authors (date reported)	Type of Institution	Prevalence Rates (%) Men	Women	Total
Mulligan and O'Grady (1971)	Psychogeriatric Units	–	–	54.0
Ingman et al. (1975)	Extended Care Facility	–	–	22.9
Christopher et al. (1978)	General/ Psychiatric Hospital Units	–	–	51.8
Salzman and Van der Kolk (1980)	General Hospital	–	–	22.6
Morgan and Gilleard (1981)	Residential Homes			33.5
Bruce (1982)	Residential Home	–	25.0	25.0
Morgan et al. (1982)	Residential Homes	32.3	34.9	34.0
Gilleard et al. (1984)	Residential Homes	–	–	35.0

– Information not reported.
Sources: Morgan (1983);[12] Gilleard et al. (1984)[17]

surveys. In the light of the evidence considered in the previous chapter high levels of hypnotic drug usage in hospitals, where both the institutional environment and the cause of admission probably contribute to sleeplessness, is not particularly surprising. In residential homes, however, the situation is a little more complex, and high levels of sleeping drug usage are not so easily accounted for.

Hypnotic drug use in residential homes. Factors which, as argued in the previous chapter, contribute to poor sleep in hospitals do not necessarily apply in residential homes. In Britain approximately 130,000 residential places for the elderly are provided under part 3 (in England and Wales) or part 4 (in Scotland) of the National Assistance Act of 1948. At least in theory these institutions are non-medical, providing care for those who 'By reason of age, infirmity, or any other circumstance are in need of care not otherwise available to them'.[13] These terms were clarified in a memorandum published by the Department of Health and Social Security in 1980 which described residential homes as being 'Primarily a means for providing a greater degree of support for those elderly people no longer able to cope with the practicalities of living in their own homes'.[14] Thus, while elderly people living in these establishments are likely to be dependent, they are much less likely to be acutely ill. A similar description would apply to those living in privately managed residential (or 'rest') homes. In the absence of noisy medical technology and staff activity, residential homes are also quieter. Furthermore, unlike hospitals where many elderly individuals are admitted only for a matter of weeks, those in residential care are likely to spend several years in this environment, ample time to become accustomed to new surroundings. Why, then, do levels of hypnotic drug usage tend to be so much higher in these homes than in the community?

In an attempt to answer this question Dr Chris Gilleard and I conducted a series of studies in local authority residential homes in Lothian Region, Scotland, between 1980 and 1984. Within this Region, which includes a large part of Edinburgh and its environs, the local authority maintained over 20 establishments providing accommodation for some 1,150 elderly people. Each resident remained under the care of a family doctor after admission, and many retained their own general practitioner. From surveys conducted in 1980,[15] 1981[16] and 1983[17] we collected detailed information on the levels of hypnotic drug use within each of these homes, and also the physical and mental status of residents, and the characteristics of the homes themselves. We then set about trying to identify factors which seemed to influence the use of sleeping drugs. The overall prevalence of sleeping drug usage found on these three occasions was 33.5, 34.0 and 35.0 per cent respectively. Levels of usage varied considerably from home to home. In one establishment, for example, over 50 per cent of the residents used hypnotics while in another, hypnotics were consumed by less than 5 per cent of the residents. We found no relationship between levels of hypnotic drug usage and the size of the home, staffing ratios within the home, sex ratios within the home, or even the proximity of the home to a main road (supposing, at the time, that noise levels from the street might be an influential factor). Nor was the likelihood of receiving a hypnotic related to the sex of the resident or the length of time they had been living in the home. However, a consistent and somewhat paradoxical relationship did emerge between hypnotic drug usage and the residents' level of dependence. As a group, the least dependent residents (i.e. those with the least degree of mental or physical impairment) showed the highest probability of receiving a hypnotic, while the likelihood of receiving hypnotics was appreciably less among the more dependent. The difference was, in fact, quite large. Comparing the two groups, the least dependent were more than twice as likely to receive sleeping drugs.

This finding could, of course, be interpreted as showing a reluctance on the part of doctors to prescribe sedative drugs for the more frail, less healthy residents. This however seems unlikely as the level of usage even among these dependent residents was much the same as that found among the elderly in the community at large, i.e. about 10 – 20 per cent. Rather, the results suggested a relative increase in usage among the fitter and less dependent, among whom levels of usage reached over 35 per cent. One possible explanation for this relationship concerns the way in which hypnotic drugs come to be prescribed in the first place. Whether in an institution or in a general practice consulting room, hypnotics are among the few drugs which are often prescribed on demand. Thus, while most physicians would not encourage requests for antibiotics, diuretics, steroids, or even vitamin tablets, it is not unprecedented for a doctor to prescribe hypnotics because the patient complains of sleeplessness and requests them. In residential homes care-staff frequently adopt the role of 'go-between', bringing the needs of the resident to the attention of their general practitioner (just as a caring relative might at home). It could be argued, therefore, that hypnotics will tend to be provided for those residents who most efficiently communicate their needs to the care staff, perhaps the least dependent and most demonstrative.[18]

There is an alternative and more controversial interpretation of these findings. Several researchers have expressed the suspicion that, in homes and hospitals for the elderly, hypnotic drugs are more likely to serve the needs of the institution than the needs of the individual resident or patient. Put more bluntly, it has been suggested that hypnotics are frequently used as a form of behavioural control, modifying sleeping patterns to suit the needs of the institution rather than the needs of the resident. In a report prepared for the United States Government and presented at the White House Conference on Aging in 1982, for example, these suspicions were echoed by Dr William Dement and others who described the use of hypnotic drugs 'in geriatric institutional settings' as 'an abomination'.[19] Strong language indeed. Could it be, then, that the needs of residential institutions discriminate between the more and the less dependent, producing differing levels of hypnotic drug usage within these two groups? Both of these interpretations rest on at least two assumptions. The first is that care staff influence prescribing, and the second assumption is that most prescriptions for hypnotics actually arise within the home. This latter point is particularly important and frequently overlooked. Just because a resident (or patient) is found to be taking sleeping tablets in an institution doesn't necessarily mean that drug usage commenced in that institution. Elderly people can be admitted to residential settings taking a variety of drugs and it could be that, in many cases, prescriptions for hypnotics actually originate outside the home.

With the consent and cooperation of Lothian Regional Social Work Department and the residential care staff, we tested the validity of both of these assumptions. To find out just how many individuals were admitted into residential care already taking hypnotic drugs we monitored all admissions into these homes for a period of six months, from March to August 1983. During this period information on hypnotic drug use and the source of admission (i.e. whether the resident was admitted from home, from hospital, etc.) was recorded by senior care staff for each new permanent resident. Table 4.4 shows some of the results from this study. Of 156 elderly people admitted to residential care during the monitoring period, 56 (35.9 per cent) were taking hypnotics on admission. Considering only the two main sources of admission (from home and from hospital), 28.6 per cent of those admitted from home were hypnotic users compared with 50 per cent of those admitted from hospital. In other words, when compared with those admitted from their own homes, those admitted from hospitals were almost twice as likely to be receiving hypnotics. Further monitoring after admission revealed that these patterns of drug usage tend to be continued within the institution. Of those taking hypnotics on admission, 85 per cent were still taking hypnotics some three

Table 4.4: Hypnotic drug usage among 156 admissions to residential care according to source of admission

	Source of admission					
	Community		Hospital		Other*	
Hypnotic users: No (%)	26	(28.6)	25	(50.0)	5	(41.7)
Non-users	65	(71.4)	25	(50.0)	7	(58.3)
Totals	91	(100.0)	50	(100.0)	12	(100.0)

* Mainly transfers from other homes.
Source: Gilleard et al. (1984)[17]

months later. However, among those who had not been taking hypnotics on admission, 29 per cent had been prescribed these drugs within three months.

In addition to the information on hypnotic drug use among new admissions we also wanted to gain some insights into the way in which hypnotics came to be prescribed in residential homes. In a series of interviews conducted by Carolien Smits,[20] general practitioners and senior care staff answered questions concerning sleep problems, and the management of sleep problems among the elderly in residential care. Most of the doctors acknowledged that sleep problems were generally brought to their attention by the care staff. Most of the care staff felt that they could discuss these problems openly and constructively with the doctors. It is interesting to note, however, that while 33 per cent of the doctors interviewed thought that some residents were unnecessarily prescribed sleeping tablets, this view was expressed by 70 per cent of the care staff. As regards the two assumptions outlined above, then, it would appear that a substantial proportion of all hypnotic drug usage did not originate within, but rather was 'inherited' by these residential homes. Furthermore, while care staff certainly did act as intermediaries between doctors and residents and did influence prescribing, there was no evidence to suggest that such influence was exercised irresponsibly. In fact, the care staff appeared to be more alarmed by the levels of sedative drug use among the residents than were the prescribers. From interviews conducted with carers and doctors only one type of prescribing emerged which might, at times, serve institutional rather than personal needs, and this practice was supported as much by the care staff as by the doctors. Asked if they thought disturbing other residents at night was a sufficient reason for prescribing someone a hypnotic, 7 out of 10 senior care staff, and 7 out of 9 general practitioners thought that it was.

There are, of course, many types of institution catering for the needs of elderly people and it cannot be assumed that all of these findings apply equally to other institutional settings. Nevertheless the study emphasised a valuable point. While high levels of hypnotic drug usage can result from over-enthusiastic prescribing, they may also result from the failure to review and withdraw drugs when they are no longer necessary. The question that remains to be answered by further research is why do some residents have their hypnotics withdrawn while others do not?

Sex differences in hypnotic drug use. One of the findings most consistently reported by the surveys shown in Table 4.2 is the presence of sex differences in hypnotic drug usage. Irrespective of when or where the studies were conducted the use of sleeping drugs is generally reported to be higher among women than among men. As can be seen from Figure 4.2, this difference between the sexes is less clearly defined in younger age groups. However, most studies report that the age-related increase in usage is more profound among women. Commenting on their results in 1962, for example, Drs McGhie and Russell observed that 'The habit of taking a hypnotic increases for both sexes with advancing years, but that both the incidence and its acceleration with age are more pronounced in the case of women.'[21] Almost 20 years later Murray and her colleagues (see Table 4.2) found a very similar pattern of usage in West London and concluded that 'The proportion of drug consumers taking an hypnotic increased with age (particularly for women)'.[22] Why, then, are elderly women more likely than their male contemporaries to receive hypnotics?

The answer to this question is far from straightforward but probably has as much to do with the social status of women as it has with the biology of sleep. Let us consider this second point first. It simply is not the case that normal age-related changes in the structure of sleep consistently affect women more than they affect men. For example, while some EEG studies report that, on average, elderly women sleep longer than elderly men, a similar number of studies have found that, on average, elderly men sleep longer than elderly women. In 1982 two Japanese researchers, Y. Hayashi and S. Endo actually reported that they had found no difference in the EEG recorded sleep of five elderly men and ten elderly women.[23] Yet sex differences in hypnotic drug usage *are* consistent, suggesting the presence of systematic and universal influences on consumption. Also consistent is the finding described in Chapter 2, that older women are more likely to report dissatisfaction with their quality of sleep than are older men. Perhaps, relative to men, women are more exposed to those circumstances which influence quality of sleep indirectly. An alternative explanation, and one still favoured in some corners of the (predominantly male) medical establishment, is that women just like to complain about things. As Ruth Cooperstock (a research worker for the Addiction Research Foundation in Toronto) found in a study of prescribing among Canadian general practitioners, the prevailing attitude among doctors was that 'Some women positively enjoy poor health.'[24] Sadly, such attitudes obscure both the issues and the evidence.

First, it has to be recognised that from a very early age little girls are encouraged to express their physical and emotional feelings of distress, while little boys are encouraged to do quite the opposite. The child is father to the man and it would not be too surprising if, in population surveys, men were less likely to admit to having problems with their sleep. On the other hand, the style of self expression encouraged in women is open to misinterpretation. Ruth Cooperstock argues convincingly that, because women are more emotionally expressive, doctors actually expect them to be more in need of mood altering drugs. The evidence also suggests that this expectation has been reinforced by the imagery of pharmaceutical advertising material which, all too often has represented women as suffering from vague emotional disorders.[25]

Against this background of cultural expectations, there are some clearly identifiable consequences of the ageing process which affect women more than men, and which are likely to result in disturbed sleep. We have already considered bereavement as an indirect influence on sleep quality in the previous chapter. In all developed countries, women tend to outlive men with the inevitable consequences that there are more widows than widowers. For example, in England and Wales estimates from the 1981 census show that for the population aged 65 and over there are more than 4 bereaved women for each bereaved man. In several of the studies shown in Table 4.2 associations between widowhood and hypnotic drug usage were reported. Drs Stevenson and Gaskell,[26] for example, found that 37 per cent of their female hypnotic users were widowed compared with only 8 per cent of the males in the same survey. In an article published in the *British Journal of Psychiatry* in 1985 Dr Colin Murray Parkes offered the following analysis of the medical profession's response to bereavement:

> Some bereaved people adopt roles which ensure that their society will be forced to accord them liminal status: they become sick, or rather they interpret the features of grief as 'symptoms' and seek help from our ritual specialists — the medical profession. Many doctors respond by writing a prescription for the bereaved person. This confirms the 'patient' in his sick role and provides him with a means to suppress some of the physiological manifestations of grief.[27]

From the research of Ann Bowling and Ann Cartwright considered in the previous chapter it is clear that these 'symptoms' are likely to include complaints of sleeplessness.[28] Allowing, then, for Dr Parkes' unfortunate choice of pronouns, it is not difficult to see how the process he describes would bias the prevalence of hypnotic drug prescribing between the sexes.

There is another consequence of outliving men. Women are more exposed to the debilitating pathologies of extreme old age and, as we saw in the previous chapter, degenerative illnesses are often associated with disturbed sleep. Thus, different levels of hypnotic drug usage between the sexes could be accounted for, at least in part, by differing levels of chronic disability. Indirect support for this possibility is provided by one of the two studies in Table 4.2 which does *not* show a sex difference in hypnotic usage. In their analysis of the prescription medicines received by 1,998 people admitted to geriatric hospitals in Britain, Professor Williamson and Dr Chopin found quite high but very similar levels of sleeping drug usage among men (22.6 per cent) and women (22.0 per cent).[29] Because this study focused on hospital admissions it is likely that levels of illness were roughly the same for both sexes and that, as a result, the need for night-time sedation was also roughly similar. This argument could also be used to explain why, in our own studies conducted in Edinburgh, we found comparable levels of hypnotic drug usage between the men and women resident in local authority accommodation.

Finally, it should not be forgotten that social custom allows men much easier access to a widely used non-prescription sedative – alcohol. In the World Health Organization's survey of 'The Elderly in Eleven Countries',[30] it was found that, whatever the local attitude towards alcohol, within each of the communities studied men consumed strong alcoholic beverages more frequently than did the women. In Britain as elsewhere, social customs may have changed considerably since the end of the Second World War, but many older people continue to subscribe to the rule that while men may enter bars alone, women may enter only if accompanied by a man. This rather biased cultural tradition limits the access of many older women to the benefits of social drinking enjoyed by men. Very little research has been conducted to assess the likely extent to which alcohol is used as a substitute for prescription sedatives or hypnotics. However, in a survey conducted in Los Angeles, California, Dr Christian Guilleminault and others found that men were more likely than women to make frequent use of alcohol as a remedy for poor sleep.[31]

In the absence of quite specific research information, accounting for the relatively greater use of hypnotic drugs by elderly women remains a matter for speculation. The evidence that is available, however, strongly suggests that sex differences in drug usage are influenced by complex interacting social processes. Certainly the issue is a lot more complicated than some of the explanations for it allow.

The frequency and duration of hypnotic drug use

Although they are informative in other respects, the prevalence rates shown in Tables 4.2 and 4.3 tell us nothing about the frequency with which hypnotic drugs are taken or the length of time for which these drugs are prescribed. Both items of information are needed if the benefits and risks of hypnotic therapy are to be assessed. For example, the risk of tolerance developing (see above) is more likely if the drug is consumed regularly over long periods of time. Important though this information is, it is surprising just how frequently it is omitted from surveys of drug use. Nevertheless, it is clear from the information that is available that many elderly people take their hypnotics on a regular basis, and that long-term use is not uncommon. Dr Ismet Karacan and his colleagues at the University of Florida, for example, found that in the age group 60 – 69 years, over 60 per cent of male hypnotic users and over 40 per cent of female hypnotic users reported taking their sleeping tablets 'often or all the time'.[32] As regards the typical duration of usage, only three of the studies shown in Table 4.2 provided this information. In all three cases the majority of hypnotic users had been taking their tablets for more than 12 months; as one author commented in the *British Medical Journal* in 1980

> Despite good intentions to the contrary, hypnotics are often prescribed for years rather than for short courses of treatment.[33]

SUMMARY

With advancing age satisfaction with sleep tends to decrease and the use of sleep promoting 'hypnotic' drugs shows a steady and reciprocal increase. While rates vary from place to place, surveys conducted in both Europe and North America suggest that sleeping tablets are regularly consumed by at least 10 per cent of the elderly population. Typically, these drugs are taken for long periods of time, even though hypnotics may lose their sleep-promoting properties after 2–3 weeks of continuous usage. Among elderly people living at home, the use of sleeping tablets is generally found to be higher among women than among men. Sex differences in sleeping drug usage can result from a number of factors. Women are more likely to experience disturbed sleep through bereavement and chronic illness, while men are more likely to use alcohol as a remedy for problem sleep. Doctors also show a greater willingness to prescribe mood altering drugs for their women patients. Among elderly people in hospitals, nursing homes, and in residential care, levels of hypnotic drug usage are particularly high. Again, rates vary from place to place but in general levels of hypnotic drug usage among institutionalised elderly people are 2 – 3 times higher than those found among the elderly at home. Most benzodiazepine hypnotics reduce sleep onset latency and intervening wakefulness, increase total sleep time, and improve personal satisfaction with sleep. However, all hypnotics become less effective with regular use.

NOTES AND REFERENCES

1. Canada Fitness Survey, 'Fitness and Aging', *Canada Fitness Survey,* 506–94 Albert Street, Ottawa (1982)

2. R. Spiegel 'Sleep and its Disorders' in M.S.J. Pathy (ed.) *Principles and Practice of Geriatric Medicine,* John Wiley and Sons Ltd, Chichester (1985) pp. 197–207

3. A full account of differences between the hypnotic trance and the state of sleep can be found in I. Oswald, *Sleep,* 4th edition, Penguin, Harmondsworth, (1980) pp. 109–23

4. See, for example, I. Oswald, 'Sleep Studies in Clinical Pharmacology', *British Journal of Clinical Pharmacology,* 10 (1980) pp. 317–26 who points out that 'Drugs that are sold for the treatment of anxiety can also be used as hypnotics'

5. E. Hartmann, *The Sleeping Pill,* Yale University Press, New Haven and London (1978)

6. D.J. Greenblatt and R. Shader, *Benzodiazepines in Clinical Practice,* Raven Press, New York (1974)

7. Details of this trial of loprazolam can be found in K. Adam, I. Oswald and C. Shapiro, 'Effects of Loprazolam and of Triazolam on Sleep and Overnight Urinary Cortisol', *Psychopharmacology,* 82 (1984) pp. 389–94

8. See K. Morgan, K. Adam and I. Oswald, 'Effects of Loprazolam and Triazolam on Psychological Functions', *Psychopharmacology,* 82 (1984) pp. 386–8

9. K. Adam, 'Are Poor Sleepers Changed into Good Sleepers by Hypnotic Drugs?' in I. Hindmarch, H. Ott, and T. Roth (eds), *Sleep, Benzodiazepines and Performance,* Springer-Verlag, Berlin (1984) pp. 44–55

10. Committee on the Review of Medicines, 'Systematic Review of the Benzodiazepines', *British Medical Journal,* 1 (1980) pp. 910–12

11. I. Oswald, C. French, K. Adam and J. Gilham, 'Benzodiazepine Hypnotics Remain Effective for 24 Weeks', *British Medical Journal,* 284 (1982) pp. 860–3

12. K. Morgan, 'Sedative-Hypnotic Drug Use and Ageing', *Archives of Gerontology and Geriatrics,* 2 (1983) pp. 181–99

13. For a description of the Act and its principal intentions see B. Watkin, *Documents on Health and Social Services 1834 to the Present Day,* Methuen and Company Limited, London (1975) pp. 94–6

14. Department of Health and Social Security, *Residential Homes for the Elderly. Arrangements for Health Care,* HMSO, London (1980)

15. K. Morgan and C.J. Gilleard, 'Patterns of Hypnotic Prescribing and Usage in Residential Homes for the Elderly', *Neuropharmacology*, 20 (1981) pp. 1355–6

16. K. Morgan, C.J. Gilleard and A. Reive, 'Hypnotic Usage in Residential Homes for the Elderly: a Prevalence and Longitudinal Analysis', *Age and Ageing*, 11 (1982) pp. 229–34

17. C.J. Gilleard, C. Smits and K. Morgan, 'Changes in Hypnotic Usage in Residential Homes for the Elderly: a Longitudinal Study', *Archives of Gerontology and Geriatrics*, 3 (1984) pp. 223–8

18. This particular view is set out in K. Morgan, 'Primary Health Care in Residential Homes for the Elderly', *British Medical Journal*, 284 (1982) p. 664

19. W.C. Dement, L.E. Miles and M.A. Carskadon, ' "White Paper" on Sleep and Ageing', *Journal of the American Geriatrics Society*, 30(1) (1982) pp. 25–50

20. C.J. Gilleard, C. Smits, K. Morgan and G. Peeters, 'Hypnotic Use Amongst Residents in Local Authority Homes for the Elderly', *Final Report to the Social Worker Services Group*, Scottish Education Department, Edinburgh (1984)

21. A. McGhie and S.M. Russell, 'The Subjective Assessment of Normal Sleep Patterns', *Journal of Mental Science*, 108 (1962) pp. 642–54

22. J. Murray, G. Dunn, P. Williams and A. Tarnapolsky, 'Factors Affecting the Consumption of Psychotropic Drugs', *Psychological Medicine*, 11 (1981) pp. 551–60

23. Y. Hayashi and S. Endo, 'All-Night Sleep Polygraphic Recordings of Healthy Aged Persons: REM and Slow Wave Sleep', *Sleep*, 5 (1982) pp. 277–83

24. R. Cooperstock, 'Sex Differences in the Use of Mood Modifying Drugs: An Explanatory Model', *Journal of Health and Social Behavior*, 12 (1971) pp. 288–44

25. R. Cooperstock, 'Some Factors Involved in the Increasing Prescribing of Psychotropic Drugs' in P. Williams and A. Clare (eds) *Psychosocial Disorders in General Practice*, Academic Press, London (1979) pp. 161–74

26. P. Stevenson and P.G. Gaskell, 'The Prescribing of Hypnotics in an Urban Practice', *Journal of the Royal College of General Practitioners*, 21 (1971) pp. 529–34

27. C.M. Parkes, 'Bereavement', *British Journal of Psychiatry*, 146, (1985) pp. 11–17

28. A. Bowling and A. Cartwright, *Life After A Death. A Study of the Elderly Widowed*, Tavistock Publications, London (1982)

29. J. Williamson and J.M. Chopin, 'Adverse Reactions to Prescribed Drugs in the Elderly: A Multicentre Investigation', *Age and Ageing*, 9 (1980) pp. 73–80

30. E. Heikkinen, W.E. Waters and Z.J. Brzezinski, *The Elderly in Eleven Countries. A Sociomedical Survey*, World Health Organization Regional Office for Europe, Copenhagen, (1983) pp. 81–2 and Figures 15 and 16

31. C. Guilleminault, R. Spiegel and W.C. Dement, 'A propos des

Insomnies', *Confront. Psychiatr.*, 15 (1977) 151–72

32. I. Karacan, J.I. Thornby, M. Anch, C.E. Holzer, G.J. Warheit, J.J. Schwab and R.L. Williams, 'Prevalence of Sleep Disturbance in a Primarily Urban Florida County', *Social Science and Medicine*, 10 (1976) pp. 239–44

33. Anonymous, 'Hypnotics and Hangover', *British Medical Journal*, 1 (1980) p. 743

34. M. Lader, 'Pharmacokinetics of the benzodiazepines: clinical implications', in G.D. Burrows (ed.) *Advances in Neuropsychopharmacology*, Libbey (1983)

35. A. Huggett, R.J. Flanagan, P. Cooke, P. Crome and D. Corless, 'Chlormethiazole and Temazepam', *British Medical Journal*, 282 (1981) p. 475

36. M. Humpel, V. Illi, W. Milius, H. Wendt and M. Kurowski, 'The pharmacokinetics and biotransformation of a new benzodiazepine (lormetazepam) in humans, 1. Absorption, distribution, elimination and metabolism of lormetazepam-5-14 C', *European Journal of Drug Metabolism and Pharmacokinetics*, 4 (1979) pp. 237–43

37. M. Humpel, B. Nieuweboer, W. Milius, H. Hanke and H. Wendt, 'Kinetics and biotransformation of lormetazepam. ii. Radioimmunologic determinations in plasma and urine of young and elderly subjects: first-pass effect', *Clinical Pharmacology and Therapeutics*, 28 (1980) pp. 673–9

38. R. Jochemsen, C.J. van Boxtel, J. Hermans and D.D. Breimer, 'Pharmacokinetics of 5 benzodiazepine hypnotics in the same panel of healthy subjects', in R. Jochemsen (ed.) *Clinical Pharmacokinetics of Benzodiazepine Hypnotics*, J.H. Pasmans, BV, 's-Gravenhage (1983) pp. 81–94

39. R. Jochemsen, P.A. van Rijn, T.G.M. Hazelzet, C.J. van Boxtel and D.D. Breimer, 'Comparative pharmacokinetics of midazolam and loprazolam in healthy subjects after oral administration', in R. Jochemsen (ed.) *Clinical Pharmacokinetics of Benzodiazepine Hypnotics*, J.H. Pasmans, BV, 's-Gravenhage (1983) pp. 176–83

5

Problems with Hypnotic Drugs

From the evidence considered in the previous chapter it is clear that the prescribing of hypnotics has become a well-established medical response to complaints of poor sleep among the elderly. In Britain, for example, it is likely that more than half a million people over the age of 65 take a sleeping drug each night.[1] Assessed simply in terms of deaths per year attributable to their use, benzodiazepines, the drug group to which most modern hypnotics belong, have proved to be remarkably safe. Without the additional assistance of alcohol or some other drug taken at the same time it is, as Ernest Hartmann points out in his book *The Sleeping Pill*, 'Almost impossible to die from an overdose of benzodiazepines'.[2] Furthermore, when taken in clinically recommended doses these drugs do not seem to cause serious physical damage and, in the long term, show 'Infinitely fewer adverse effects than alcohol or tobacco'.[3] In essence, then, benzodiazepine sedative-hypnotics are probably the least toxic of all currently prescribed psychotropic drugs, and the least poisonous sleeping drugs ever marketed. There is, however, much more to the safety of hypnotics than their potential for causing physical illness or lethal damage when taken chronically or in overdose. As mentioned in the previous chapter, drugs used to induce sleep exert a powerful influence on mood and behaviour; such drugs have the potential, therefore, to affect not only physical but also psychological wellbeing. Throughout the discussion which follows effects on behaviour, mood, and mental processes will be considered as 'psychological' effects.

Interest in the psychological impact of hypnotics was greatly stimulated by laboratory studies which showed that sleeping drugs (whether barbiturate or benzodiazepine) taken at night can adversely affect the efficiency of behaviour the following day. In 1971, for example, A.J. Walters and Dr (now Professor) Malcolm Lader reported that in healthy young volunteers, performance on some psychological tests, for instance the speed of key tapping, was impaired up to 12 hours after either a single 10 mg dose of nitrazepam, or a 200 mg dose of butobarbitone sodium (a once popular barbiturate hypnotic).[4] Research into the behavioural consequences of hypnotic drug usage gathered momentum throughout the 1970s, and continues to augment the attention paid to the efficacy and toxicity of these drugs. As a result, it is now widely recognised that in addition to their desirable effects, even the apparently innocuous benzodiazepine hypnotics can have extremely undesirable effects on mood, on daytime behaviour, and even on sleep itself. In the sections which follow these unwanted effects will be considered using examples selected from the research literature. This discussion will, incidentally, focus almost exclusively on benzodiazepine drugs. In Britain as elsewhere, barbiturate and other non-benzodiazepine hypnotics are now infrequently prescribed.

RESIDUAL EFFECTS AND DRUG ACCUMULATION

Ideally, hypnotics should be active only during the hours of sleep. As demonstrated by the experiments of Walters and Lader, and since by many others, this apparently simple requirement is not always met and the sedative action of some hypnotics can persist long after waking, influencing and disrupting daytime activities. Various terms have been used to describe these effects, including 'hangover effects', 'residual sequelae', and 'residual effects'. The term 'residual effects' will be used here; 'hangover' is a little inaccurate as it traditionally refers to the consequences of drug *withdrawal* (as with alcohol) rather than drug persistence, while the more elegant 'sequelae' causes too many problems with pronunciation.

Residual effects can be additive. It was noted in Chapter 4 that drugs with a long half-life tend to remain active in the body longer than drugs with a shorter half-life. Some hypnotics persist for so long that traces of the drug are still present at the following bedtime. If such a hypnotic is taken on two consecutive nights, peak concentrations of the second dose will be added to residual concentrations of the first, leading to even higher residual concentrations the next day. In this way residual amounts of the drug can accumulate so that daytime behaviour perhaps unaffected after a single dose can be affected after several consecutive doses.

These residual effects arising from sleeping drug usage have long been recognised. In an essay 'On the Use of Hypnotic Drugs in the Treatment of Insomnia' published in the *Journal of Mental Science* in 1905, Dr W. Maule Smith identified one of the main characteristics of drug induced sleep as being 'The inability of the parts acted upon by the drug to free themselves from the enforced restraint due to the lingering effect of the hypnotic'. The perspicacious Dr Smith went on to note that 'The degree of this effect varies with the constitution of the drug and the dose prescribed'.[5] The additional influence of age, however, is omitted from this observation. As mentioned in the previous chapter, ageing bodies become less efficient at clearing drugs from the system. In elderly users, therefore, hypnotics tend to persist longer, and daytime behavioural disruptions due to the 'lingering' effects of these drugs become more likely. In addition, residual drug effects in the elderly may be super-imposed upon existing age-dependent reductions in mental and physical efficiency. Consequently, among elderly users residual effects are not only more likely, but can also be more profound. Both of these points can be illustrated with reference to nitrazepam which was one of the first benzodiazepine hypnotics to be introduced.

A relatively long-acting drug, nitrazepam has a half-life in the range 20 – 40 hours (see Table 4.1) and is generally prescribed in either 5 mg or 10 mg doses. In 1972 Professor J. Grimley Evans and Dr E.H. Jarvis of Newcastle General Hospital described a state of mental confusion in frail elderly patients which they attributed to the cumulative effects of nitrazepam taken in normal therapeutic doses.[6] This distressing confusional state which, they suggested, could be mistaken for dementia, subsided when the drug was withdrawn. In 1978 the Boston Collaborative Drug Surveillance Program (an international drug monitoring project) published results from a survey of 2,111 hospitalised inpatients of all ages who had received nitrazepam, and whose level of daytime drowsiness and sedation had been assessed by specially trained nurses. Among those receiving a 10 mg dose, the frequency of unwanted daytime sedation increased steadily with age. Fifty-five per cent of those aged over 80 were judged to be excessively drowsy during the day. Again, drug accumulation was one of the reasons suggested for these unwanted effects.[7]

Not all residual effects are so easily observed. As already suggested, hypnotics can cause subtle changes in behaviour which, although not apparent to the casual observer, can be detected using carefully administered psychological tests. Such tests may indicate that reaction times are slowed, that judgement is impaired, or that caution is reduced, even though the individual concerned experiences no subjective impairment. Thus, while some of the tasks employed to detect residual effects may seem irrelevant to everyday behaviour, the findings from such procedures have very real implications for the daytime efficiency of hypnotic users. In a study reported in 1977, Dr C.M. Castleden and others at the University of Southampton found that in a group of healthy elderly volunteers, performance on a simple pencil and paper test (deleting every occurrence of the letter 'e' from a page of prose) was still impaired 36 hours after taking nitrazepam in a single 10 mg dose.[8] In the same study, however, the test performance of younger subjects appeared to be unaffected by the drug at this time. The researchers concluded that, even after single doses, the elderly appear to be more sensitive to the residual effects of nitrazepam.

These clinical and experimental findings clearly illustrate the residual and cumulative effects of long-acting hypnotic drugs in elderly users. The severity of these effects, which range from deficits on psychological tests, through overt daytime drowsiness, to states of mental confusion, doubtless depends upon the constitution of the individual as well as the duration of drug usage. While frail elderly people appear particularly vulnerable to cumulative effects following multiple doses, healthy elderly people can be adversely affected by just a single dose. Other long-acting hypnotic drugs have shown a similar tendency to disrupt daytime performance in older users. For example, in studies conducted in Edinburgh, 21 consecutive nightly doses of flurazepam 30 mg were found to progressively impair the performance of middle-aged volunteers on laboratory tests of concentration and memory. On the same tests, however, performance was unimpaired following consecutive nightly doses of the shorter acting drugs lormetazepam,[9] loprazolam, and triazolam.[10]

Interestingly, however, nitrazepam remained one of the most popularly prescribed hypnotics for the elderly (at least in Britain) until the early 1980s. One of the reasons for this was undoubtedly the widespread but at that time untested assumption that residual effects from long-acting drugs could be effectively controlled by employing lower doses. For example, from the surveys of hypnotic drug use conducted in Edinburgh between 1980 and 1984 (and described in the previous chapter) we found that nitrazepam was most often prescribed for elderly patients in the lower (5 mg) dose, as opposed to the higher (10 mg) dose. Two research questions arise here. First, in elderly users are the residual and cumulative effects associated with nitrazepam significantly offset by using a lower dose? And second, in terms of residual and cumulative effects, how does low-dose nitrazepam compare with a shorter acting drug?

With the help of 12 volunteers aged between 75 and 96 I attempted to answer these questions by comparing the residual effects of nitrazepam taken in a 5 mg dose with those of a shorter acting benzodiazepine, lormetazepam (which has a half-life of 13 – 14 hours; see Table 4.1), taken in a 1 mg dose.[11] It will be remembered from Chapter 4 that lormetazepam is a more potent benzodiazepine than nitrazepam and that in terms of hypnotic efficacy a 1 mg dose of the former drug is roughly equivalent to a 5 mg dose of the latter. In a double-blind study both hypnotics, and a placebo, were taken for seven consecutive nights. On selected mornings throughout the study volunteers were assessed on a simple 'reciprocal tapping' test which was conducted as follows. Using a stylus each volunteer was asked to tap alternately two circular targets placed 25 cm (about 10 inches) apart as quickly and as accurately as possible for 30 seconds. Contact with either of the targets registered electronically as a 'hit', while contact with any other part of the apparatus registered as an 'error'. As with many real life situations (for example, typing or knitting) this test requires a 'trade-off' between speed and accuracy. Too much speed will increase errors, while too much caution will reduce speed. In accordance with the test instructions, therefore, volunteers select a level of performance which attempts to maximise both. Accuracy on the test was measured by the total number of errors expressed as a percentage of all taps. Thus, an error score of 10 per cent

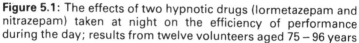

Figure 5.1: The effects of two hypnotic drugs (lormetazepam and nitrazepam) taken at night on the efficiency of performance during the day; results from twelve volunteers aged 75 – 96 years

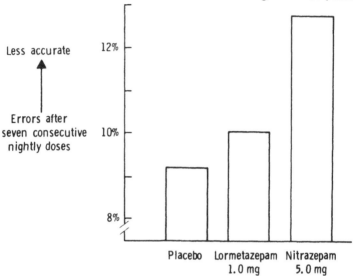

Note: These results are from a 'reciprocal tapping' test; volunteers were required to tap alternately two circular targets placed 25 cm apart as quickly and as accurately as possible for 30 seconds. Four different sizes of target were used (from 2 to 6 cm in diameter) and were presented first in ascending order, then in descending order of size. 'Errors' are the average percentage of taps which missed the target (irrespective of size). Source: Data from Morgan, Effects of Repeated Dose Nitrazepam and Lormetazepam on Psychomotor Performance in the Elderly, *Psychopharmacology*, Vol. 86 (1985) pp. 209–11

would mean that 1 in 10 taps actually missed the intended target.

After a single dose, neither drug seemed to impair accuracy on the tapping task. After seven consecutive doses, however, performance associated with nitrazepam was much less accurate than that following lormetazepam or the placebo, a result consistent with the gradual accumulation of the longer acting drug (see Figure 5.1). It is interesting that nitrazepam was not associated with a reduction in the *speed* of tapping, suggesting that the drug actually reduced caution; after all, accuracy could have been maintained simply by slowing down! Perhaps these elderly volunteers did not realise that their performance was impaired and consequently made no attempt to compensate for their reduced accuracy. Whatever the underlying cause of the deficit, the implications are clear. Even in low doses, repeated use of long-acting benzodiazepines poses a threat to the daytime efficiency of elderly people.

While residual and cumulative effects have been demonstrated in the first few days or weeks of hypnotic drug consumption, there is some evidence that, after very prolonged use, these unwanted residual effects may diminish. In a study reported by Dr Cameron Swift and his colleagues at the University of Dundee, little evidence of 'unwanted sedation, confusion, or unsteadiness' was found among 253 long-term elderly nitrazepam and flurazepam users, some of whom had been taking these drugs for up to 15 years.[12] By the time such tolerance has had time to develop, however, the individual is likely to have become drug dependent, a problem discussed later in this chapter.

The impact of hypnotic drugs on daytime performance in the elderly is, at present, under researched and ill understood. As explained in Chapter 1, laboratory studies evaluating the effects of sleeping tablets have, until quite recently, been conducted mainly among young adults, and a lot more needs to be learned about residual effects among the elderly both inside and outside the laboratory. Certainly, the 'real' impact of these drugs is likely to be extremely complex, particularly where residual effects interact with existing age-related risk factors. Even without hypnotics elderly people are, relative to younger adults, more likely to fall over,[13] have accidents in the home,[14] and experience forgetfulness and disorientation. As yet, little systematic research has been conducted into how these events may be influenced by sleeping drug usage. It should also be kept in mind that residual effects may be amplified or otherwise complicated by the concomitant use of drugs which, like hypnotics, act on the central nervous system (for example pain-killers, tranquillisers, anti-depressants and, of course, alcohol). Multiple drug use is not uncommon in old age; in the Edinburgh surveys described in the previous chapter, over 25 per cent of elderly hypnotic drug users were concomitantly receiving centrally acting medications during the day.[15]

REBOUND EFFECTS

Rebound insomnia. It was mentioned in Chapter 3 that psychotropic drugs can affect the body not only when they are present, but also when they are withdrawn. Again, alcohol provides a good example of this; taken in large amounts, its presence may be associated with feelings of wellbeing, while its withdrawal may be accompanied by the malaise of hangover. Most of the remaining problems to be discussed in this chapter concern withdrawal effects. Before discussing these, we will first reconsider a related issue which was briefly mentioned in Chapter 4.

Regular hypnotic usage is associated with tolerance, whereby the body becomes accustomed to the drug, larger doses of which are then needed in order to achieve the original effect. In practice, larger doses are not usually taken and the sleep inducing properties of the same repeated dose consequently diminish over time. Tolerance indicates that the nervous system is undergoing certain adaptive changes to compensate for, and override the effects of the drug. Conceptually, the presence of the drug is making the body 'push' much harder in the direction of greater sleeplessness in order to maintain its usual level of functioning. Dose by dose the pressure behind this 'push' increases until, as is sometimes the case with hypnotics and tranquillisers, the effects of the drug are largely negated. If a drug to which tolerance has developed is abruptly withdrawn, then all resistance to these adaptive changes is removed, and what was compensation in the presence of the drug becomes overcompensation in its absence. Following regular usage, therefore, withdrawal of benzodiazepine drugs is followed by a characteristic disturbance of sleep referred to as 'rebound insomnia'.

The onset and severity of rebound effects will depend upon the speed at which the drug is eliminated from the body. Thus, the withdrawal of shorter acting drugs produces an earlier rebound than the withdrawal of long acting drugs. Indeed, some very long acting drugs like flurazepam take so long to leave the system that rebound effects are actually minimised.[9] In such cases the notion of 'abrupt' withdrawal is, perhaps, inappropriate. Figure 5.2, for example, compares the effects of loprazolam 1 mg and triazolam 0.5 mg on the average amount of wakefulness intervening during the sleep of 9 middle-aged

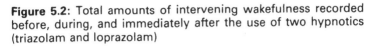

Figure 5.2: Total amounts of intervening wakefulness recorded before, during, and immediately after the use of two hypnotics (triazolam and loprazolam)

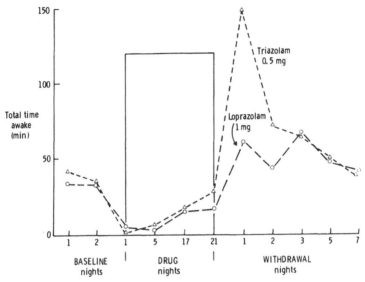

TOTAL MINUTES OF WAKEFULNESS ACCUMULATED AFTER THE FIRST ONSET OF SLEEP
(Each point is the average for 9 middle-aged volunteers)

Note: Placebo (dummy) tablets were taken during the 'baseline' and 'withdrawal' periods.
Source: Adam *et al.*, *Psychopharmacology*, Vol. 82 (1984) pp. 389–94.

volunteers (for loprazolam, this information was considered in Figure 4.3). EEG recordings of sleep made on five consecutive 'withdrawal' nights (during which placebos were substituted for the active hypnotics) show that wakefulness increased dramatically in the absence of the drugs. It is also clear that maximum levels of wakefulness were reached much earlier, and were also more intense, following the withdrawal of the shorter acting triazolam. Nevertheless the body adjusts and, after seven nights, levels of intervening wakefulness returned to the pre-drug (baseline) levels.

REM rebound. Hypnotics also affect the overall structure of sleep, reducing total amounts of both REM and stage 4 sleep. On withdrawal of the drug REM sleep can also rebound, sometimes to well above its pre-drug level. As dreams are most

107

likely to occur during the REM stage, this rebound can be associated with vivid dreaming and sometimes nightmares. Once again, the rebound effect subsides as the body re-adjusts to the absence of the drug.

Rebound anxiety. It was mentioned in the previous chapter that in addition to promoting and maintaining sleep, hypnotics also reduce anxiety. In fact, hypnotic and tranquillising drugs are virtually identical. Where poor sleep is accompanied by stress a long-acting hypnotic drug may be prescribed especially to exploit its residual anti-anxiety effects during the day. With repeated usage tolerance to these tranquillising effects also develops such that, on withdrawal, anxiety can 'rebound' above pre-drug levels.

Although they are transient, rebound effects have serious implications for successful withdrawal. For those who wish to discontinue their hypnotics but who are unaware of, or unable to cope with, the immediate consequences, a short period of rebound insomnia accompanied perhaps by increased daytime anxiety may be enough to convince them that they need their sleeping tablets after all. In this way many people may continue to take their hypnotics not to promote sleep *per se*, but rather to avoid the unpleasant consequences of withdrawal. This will be considered in greater detail when we consider drug dependence.

DAYTIME WITHDRAWAL

In response to growing concern over the unwanted daytime effects of long-acting drugs like nitrazepam and flurazepam, shorter acting, but equally effective hypnotics were developed and introduced. On theoretical grounds benzodiazepines with a relatively short half-life are less likely to be associated with residual effects, and unlikely to accumulate with repeated doses. In practice, this would appear to be the case, as Figure 5.1 demonstrates. Paradoxically, however, there is a disguised advantage in the regular use of longer acting benzodiazepines, and this advantage lies in their ability to postpone daytime withdrawal effects. As already mentioned, withdrawal effects occur when concentrations of a tolerated drug fall below a critical level. Usually, this happens when the drug is actually discontinued, resulting in (among other things) the rebound

Figure 5.3: Daily ratings of anxiety during, and after the use of two hypnotics (triazolam and loprazolam)

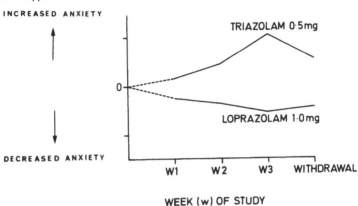

Source: Data from Morgan and Oswald, 'Anxiety caused by a Short-Life Hypnotic', *British Medical Journal*, Vol. 284 (1982) p. 942.

insomnia and anxiety described above. As hypnotic drug concentrations decline as each dose is metabolised and cleared, withdrawal effects may also occur between doses, i.e. during the day. However, significant daytime withdrawal is unlikely to accompany the use of longer acting hypnotics since, if regularly taken, there is always a residual amount of drug present in the body. This is not the case with some *very* short acting drugs which may be completely eliminated long before the next dose is taken. As a result, rebound anxiety may emerge during the day as drug concentrations fall.

Evidence of daytime withdrawal effects associated with a very short acting hypnotic unexpectedly came to light in the laboratory trials of loprazolam and triazolam to which reference has already been made. Both drugs were consumed for 21 consecutive nights, after which, and unbeknownst to the volunteers, placebos were substituted for the active hypnotics and the effects of withdrawal were observed. Throughout this period all the volunteers were asked to rate each evening how anxious they had felt on that day. Ratings were made by placing a mark on a 10 cm visual analogue scale between the statements 'terrible agitation' and 'utterly calm and peaceful'.

The results from this simple exercise are shown in Figure 5.3. The progressive decrease in reported daytime anxiety associated with loprazolam is typical for long and intermediate half-life benzodiazepine hypnotics (see Table 4.1). The pattern of self-rated anxiety associated with triazolam is quite different. As tolerance to this *very* short acting drug developed with repeated use, levels of daytime anxiety and agitation actually increased.[16] For both hypnotics, these effects subsided when the drugs were withdrawn. Similar findings have since been reported from other laboratories. In two separate studies in which the very short acting hypnotics midazolam and triazolam were taken on 7 and 14 consecutive nights respectively, Dr Anthony Kales and his colleagues at Pennsylvania State University found that both drugs increased levels of daytime anxiety in their chronic insomniac volunteers.[17] Furthermore, EEG recordings from these studies showed that after 7 or more nights of continuous usage both drugs caused increased wakefulness in the early hours of the morning. This interesting effect was attributed to the rapid elimination of the hypnotics during the night which, once tolerance had developed, resulted in a rebound 'early morning insomnia' during the last 2 hours of sleep. It should be noted that in both Kales' study, and in the Edinburgh trials described above, triazolam was consumed in a 0.5 mg dose. The maximum dose now recommended for this drug in the United Kingdom is 0.25 mg.

DRUG DEPENDENCE

The effects of abrupt withdrawal so far considered have been those associated with relatively short-term hypnotic drug use (i.e. 1 – 3 weeks). While clearly undesirable these rebound effects on mood and sleep seem to be largely unpleasant but tolerable. After longer periods of use in excess of say, 4 – 6 months, the consequences of abruptly discontinuing the drug become more severe and more distressing. As a result, some people come to depend on their hypnotics not to improve their sleep quality but rather to avoid the consequences of withdrawal. At this point a state of physical drug dependency has been achieved. In addition, the consumption of a sleeping tablet can, over a long period of time, become part of a nightly 'going to bed' ritual and, like many ritual behaviours, its performance may inspire feelings of security and comfort. To neglect or even to think about neglecting such rituals can produce feelings of apprehension and, in some cases, utter panic. Not infrequently, this psychological need to take the drug combines with, and is strengthened by physical dependency. Among chronic benzo-diazepine users, elements of both physical and psychological dependency often co-exist.[18]

It is only in recent years that the consequences of long-term benzodiazepine use have received research (and latterly media) attention. It now has to be recognised that dependency is one of the major problems associated with protracted benzodiazepine use. As already noted, long-term use is by no means exceptional among elderly hypnotic users, many of whom may be supporting a drug 'habit' rather than positively improving the quality of their sleep. For example, in a survey conducted in a single general practice in West Lothian, Scotland, it was found that over half of all elderly patients receiving hypnotics had been regular users for more than 3 years.[19] Most of these patients expressed a desire to discontinue their hypnotics, and many reported that they had tried to do so. When asked why they continued to take sleeping tablets, however, 68 per cent of all the users replied that they could not sleep without them. After such long-term drug use this sleeplessness was most likely a feature of the severe rebound referred to as the 'withdrawal' or 'abstinence' syndrome.

Among long-term users (and, very occasionally, among shorter term users) abrupt benzodiazepine withdrawal can be accompanied by a syndrome which, as described by the Committee on the Review of Medicines, can include 'anxiety, apprehension, tremor, insomnia, nausea and vomiting'.[20] Summarising the available research evidence in 1983 Dr Hannes Petursson and Professor Malcolm Lader concluded that, when benzodiazepine treatment is discontinued, such withdrawal symptoms can be anticipated in 24 – 45 per cent of those who have taken their drugs for 2 – 4 years, and in 75 per cent of those who have consumed benzodiazepines for 6 – 8 years.[18] In a study reported in 1981, Petursson and Lader showed that, in a group of long-term predominantly young tranquilliser users whose daily intake was first halved for two weeks, and then discontinued altogether, withdrawal symptoms were maximum after 3 – 7 days, but subsided after 2 – 4 weeks. All of these individuals reported a marked rebound insomnia, some getting less than 2 – 3 hours of sleep per night in the first few days of withdrawal. After 10 days, however, duration of sleep had returned to normal (i.e. pre-withdrawal) levels.[21] [As mentioned in the previous chapter, the difference between benzodiazepine tranquillisers and benzodiazepine hypnotics is largely semantic. While current research focuses on tranquilliser dependence, the results from such research also apply to the long-term use of hypnotics.]

Drug withdrawal of the type described by Dr Petursson and Professor Lader requires a great deal of motivation and stamina on the part of the drug user. At present it remains a matter of conjecture whether many elderly hypnotic drug users have the physical or emotional resources at their disposal to confront and overcome a 'problem' which they may be unaware of, or at least quite prepared to live with. Clearly, the best solution all round would be to prevent such dependence occurring in the first place by vigorously discouraging long-term use.

Non-benzodiazepine hypnotics

As mentioned at the beginning of this chapter, the bulk of all prescribed hypnotics are benzodiazepines. Nevertheless, non-benzodiazepine and non-barbiturate hypnotics continue to be prescribed. Because of their consistent use amongst the elderly, two of these drugs merit some attention here.

In Britain *dichloralphenazone*, a derivative of chloral hydrate (one of the first synthetic hypnotics), is not infrequently prescribed for elderly people living at home.[19] While there is no research evidence to suggest that it is any more effective or any safer than available benzodiazepines, dichloralphenazone has long enjoyed a reputation for being a 'safe and satisfactory hypnotic of first choice' for the treatment of poor sleep in elderly patients.[6] Unfortunately, this drug has a low therapeutic index, which means that the difference between the effective dose and the fatal overdose is not great (the effective dose being 600 mg to 1.2 g while the average fatal dose is about 10 g). Dichloralphenazone can cause excessive intestinal flatulence, and is known to be a drug of dependence.

In contrast to dichloralphenazone, *chlormethiazole* is rarely prescribed for the elderly living at home, but is commonly prescribed as a hypnotic for elderly hospital inpatients.[22] While it has been reported that daytime behaviour in the elderly is unaffected after a single night-time dose of this drug,[23] the behavioural impact of repeated doses has not been thoroughly investigated. Chlormethiazole is also a drug of dependence, though as it tends to be used in controlled hospital environments this cannot be viewed as a major problem. Again, there is no experimental evidence to suggest that chlormethiazole is a more effective or safer hypnotic than available and better researched intermediate half-life benzodiazepines.

SUMMARY

While safe and effective in the treatment of problem sleep, benzodiazepine hypnotics are associated with a variety of unwanted side-effects. Because of age-related changes in the way the body responds to and handles drugs, and also because of the widespread long-term use of sleeping tablets amongst older people, many of these unwanted effects are more likely and tend to be more profound in the elderly. Long-acting drugs produce residual and cumulative effects which, among elderly people, can include covert reductions in behavioural efficiency, overt daytime drowsiness, and sometimes mental confusion. Such effects are considerably less likely with shorter acting hypnotics. However, while devoid of residual action, repeated doses of *very* short acting sleeping drugs are associated with daytime withdrawal effects and can significantly increase levels of daytime anxiety. Most hypnotics produce a characteristic 'rebound' when discontinued after even a brief period (1 – 3 weeks) of regular use. The shorter acting the hypnotic, the earlier and the more intense the rebound effects, which can include sleeplessness, anxiety, and vivid, sometimes disturbing dreams. In all age groups the long-term use of hypnotics carries the risk of dependence, as evidenced by the emergence of upleasant withdrawal symptoms when the drug is discontinued. Long-term use, however, appears to be extremely common among elderly people. Many elderly hypnotic users are also taking accompanying medication which can increase the risk of behavioural or intellectual disturbance from sleeping drugs.

NOTES AND REFERENCES

1. This figure is conservatively estimated (on the basis of the

prevalence rates discussed in Chapter 4) as 5 per cent of the current elderly population of 8 million

2. E. Hartmann, *The Sleeping Pill*, Yale University Press, New Haven and London (1978) p. 21

3. J. Marks, *The Benzodiazepines. Use, Overuse, Misuse, Abuse*, 2nd Edition, MTP Press Ltd, Lancaster (1985)

4. A.J. Walters and M.H. Lader, 'Hangover Effects of Hypnotics in Man', *Nature*, 229 (1971) pp. 637–8

5. W.M. Smith, 'On the Use of Hypnotic Drugs in the Treatment of Insomnia', *Journal of Mental Science*, 51 (1905) pp. 561–75

6. J.G. Evans and E.H. Jarvis, 'Nitrazepam and the Elderly', *British Medical Journal*, 4 (1972) p. 487

7. D.J. Greenblatt and M.D. Allen, 'Toxicity of Nitrazepam in the Elderly: A Report from the Boston Collaborative Drug Surveillance Program', *British Journal of Clinical Pharmacology*, 5 (1978) pp. 407–13

8. C.M. Castleden, C.F. George, D. Marcer and C. Hallett, 'Increased Sensitivity to Nitrazepam in Old Age', *British Medical Journal*, 1 (1977) pp. 10–12

9. I. Oswald, K. Adam, S. Borrow and C. Idzikowski, 'The Effects of Two Hypnotics on Sleep, Subjective Feelings and Skilled Performance', in P. Passouant and I. Oswald (eds) *Pharmacology of the States of Alertness*, Pergamon Press, Oxford and New York (1979)

10. K. Morgan, K. Adam and I. Oswald, 'Effects of Loprazolam and of Triazolam on Psychological Functions', *Psychopharmacology*, 82 (1984) pp. 386–8

11. K. Morgan, 'Effects of Repeated Dose Nitrazepam and Lormetazepam on Psychomotor Performance in the Elderly', *Psychopharmacology*, 86 (1985) pp. 209–11

12. C.G. Swift, M.R. Swift, J. Hamley, I.H. Stevenson and J. Crooks, 'Side-Effect "Tolerance" in Elderly Long-Term Recipients of Benzodiazepine Hypnotics', *Age and Ageing*, 13 (1984) pp. 335–43

13. For a review of this topic see P.W. Overstall, 'Falls', in M.S.J. Pathy (ed.) *Principles and Practice of Geriatric Medicine*, John Wiley and Sons, Chichester (1985)

14. See Age Concern, *Profiles of the Elderly 5: Accidents*, Age Concern (England) Research Publications, Mithcham, Surrey (1977)

15. K. Morgan, C.J. Gilleard and A. Reive, 'Hypnotic Usage in Residential Homes for the Elderly', *Age and Ageing*, 11 (1982) pp. 229–34

16. K. Morgan and I. Oswald, 'Anxiety Caused By a Short-Life Hypnotic', *British Medical Journal*, 284 (1984) p. 942

17. A. Kales, C.R. Soldatos, E.O. Bixler and J.D. Kales, 'Early Morning Insomnia with Rapidly Eliminated Benzodiazepines', *Science*, (1983) pp. 95–7

18. H. Petursson and M.H. Lader, *Dependence on Tranquillizers*, Maudsley Monograph Volume 28, Oxford University Press, Oxford (1984)

19. D. Hay, R.M. Milne and C.J. Gilleard, 'Hypnotic Drugs, Old People and Their Habits: A General Practice Study', *Health Bulletin*,

44 (4) (1986) pp. 218–22

20. Committee on the Review of Medicines, 'Systematic Review of the Benzodiazepines', *British Medical Journal*, 280 (1980) pp. 910–12

21. H. Petursson and M.H. Lader, 'Withdrawal from Long-Term Benzodiazepine Treatment', *British Medical Journal*, 283 (1981) pp. 643–5

22. C.J. Gilleard and K. Morgan, 'Hypnotic Usage in the Elderly in Residential Care: Edinburgh (Lothian Region) and Islington Surveys', in A.N. Nicholson (ed.) *Hypnotics in Clinical Practice*, The Medicine Publishing Foundation, Oxford (1982)

23. R.S. Briggs, C.M. Castleden and C.A. Kraft, 'Improved Hypnotic Treatment Using Chlormethiazole and Temazepam', *British Medical Journal*, 279 (1980) pp. 601–4

6

Alternatives to Hypnotic Drugs

In guidelines published in 1981 the Committee on the Review of Medicines recommended that 'The use of benzodiazepine therapy in the elderly, especially use of long-acting benzodiazepines for insomnia, be undertaken for short periods of time, and only after careful consideration'.[1] Quite apart from this specific concern for the elderly, many clinical sleep researchers now agree that, irrespective of age, the most appropriate use of hypnotic drugs is in the treatment of 'transient situational insomnia'.[2] For many elderly people, however, dissatisfaction with sleep is neither transient nor situational but appears, rather, to be permanent and constitutional. Clearly, the use of hypnotic drugs in such cases is an unrealistic and wholly inappropriate response. This chapter is concerned with alternative strategies for responding to, and coping with sleep problems in old age. These alternatives range from what might be termed 'common-sense advice' to some recently evaluated psychological treatments for improving sleep quality in elderly people. I would like to emphasise again that this book is not intended as a clinical manual and does not aim to provide a do-it-yourself guide to treatment. Rather, in providing this information, the aim is to inform the reader of the existence of rational non-pharmacological approaches to the management of insomnia, and to explore the opportunities for self-help in the control of sleep problems. This discussion will repeatedly bring us into contact with the notion of insomnia and it would be helpful, therefore, if we first considered what is meant by this term.

WHAT IS INSOMNIA?

One of the major problems in defining insomnia is the absence of a clear one-to-one relationship between the objective characteristics of sleep, and the subjective complaint of poor sleep. For example some people who consistently complain of poor quality sleep show no signs of EEG sleep disturbance.[3] On the other hand, some people whose sleep appears from the EEG to be excessively short (so called 'healthy insomniacs') awake feeling well-rested and content.[4] Often, then, complaints of insomnia reflect the individual's *experience* of sleep rather than those characteristics of sleep observed by the researcher. While most researchers and clinicians seem to agree on this point, opinions differ as to whether the complaint of poor sleep is a sufficient or even a necessary condition for defining insomnia. For example, Professor Ian Oswald, emphasising the subjective nature of insomnia, states that it is not a disease but 'a symptom, a complaint' of poor sleep.[5] On the other hand, a definition which includes the objective characteristics of sleep (with or without a complaint) is preferred by Professor Anthony and Dr Joyce Kales who, in their book *Evaluation and Treatment of Insomnia* describe the condition as 'A relative lack of sleep, an inadequate quality of sleep or both'.[6]

In the present context the difference between these definitions is important. If viewed as 'relatively' short sleep, some elderly people whose sleep has changed markedly in old age might, inappropriately, be regarded as insomniacs even though they are satisfied and refreshed by the sleep they get. In the discussion which follows, then, it will be assumed that insomnia in old age includes some of the changes described in Chapter 2, together with a complaint of poor sleep. Having said that, it should also be realised that complaints about sleep are greatly influenced by expectations. Thus, advice and information which helps to foster a realistic expectation of sleep in old age, and which should accompany any professionally mediated treatment, may be sufficiently reassuring to pre-empt the need for direct therapeutic intervention.

MEDICAL TREATMENT FOR UNDERLYING CAUSES
OF INSOMNIA

As described in Chapter 3, insomnia in old age is often secondary to a medical or psychiatric disorder. Under these circumstances it is reasonable to seek treatment, not for the sleeplessness as such, but for the underlying cause. Specific treatments for arthritis, for example, can greatly relieve sleep disturbance from stiff and painful joints, while other painful conditions might be treated more appropriately with analgesic (pain killing) rather than hypnotic drugs. Similarly, antidepressant drugs, many of which possess sedative properties, can be used to treat both depression and the sleeplessness associated with it.[7]

Medical treatment can also be provided for those conditions in which sleep loss and tiredness may be the principal, and sometimes the only complaint. These include sleep apnoea, periodic movements in sleep (PMS), and night-time cramps etc. (see Chapter 3). Where sleep apnoea is associated with obesity, supervised weight reduction is, of course, essential although loss of weight can in itself lead to loss of sleep (see below). While progress in the drug treatment of sleep apnoea and PMS has been described as 'very rapid and encouraging',[8] there are as yet no widely agreed specific treatments for these disorders. There is agreement, however, that hypnotic drugs, which can further depress breathing, are counter-indicated in the treatment of sleep-related respiratory disorders. Night-time cramps, on the other hand, seem to present less of a problem for medical treatment and can be reduced in number, severity, and duration by nightly doses of quinine sulphate.[9]

As already noted, certain drugs can be the cause of insomnia and consultation with the prescribing doctor may lead to the offending item or items being substituted or discontinued. The medical assessment of a sleep problem also serves to exclude possible underlying and medically treatable causes before alternative therapies are attempted. It should be kept in mind, however, that complaints of poor sleep in the doctor's surgery may be interpreted as a request for hypnotic drugs. General practitioners are not always sure what their patients want, and may guess, sometimes wrongly. On the basis of interviews conducted with both prescribers and patients, for example, it has been estimated that while doctors suppose that over 80 per cent of their patients want a prescription, only about 30 to 50 per cent of patients actually do.[10]

Supervised drug withdrawal

Where sleeping drugs have been taken continuously for long periods of time (say, 4 – 6 months) a systematic and supervised withdrawal can help to minimise some of the unpleasant rebound effects. If consulted beforehand, the prescribing doctor can offer advice on the consequences of discontinuing a particular hypnotic, and is likely to recommend a step-wise dose reduction rather than an abrupt withdrawal. In Britain as elsewhere benzodiazepine withdrawal groups, supervised by psychologists or other health-care workers, are just beginning to confront the widespread problem of 'normal-dose' dependency described in the previous chapter. Such groups can offer both emotional support and practical help in anxiety management throughout the withdrawal period.

GOOD HABITS AND SELF-HELP

Dr Nathaniel Kleitman, one of the pioneers of sleep research, used the phrase 'hygiene of sleep' to describe collectively those personal habits and behaviours which can improve or maintain sleep quality.[11] Clinical observations and research findings have since contributed to an extensive list of 'dos' and 'don'ts' for getting the best out of sleep, and some of these are summarised below. Alone, or in combination with specific therapies, these self help measures provide a logical first step towards improving satisfaction with sleep in old age.

Regularity and sleep

It was emphasised in Chapter 2 that sleep and wakefulness are, by and large, synchronised with the 24-hour day, a result of the internal or biological 'clock' becoming entrained by the external zeitgebers like mealtimes, work routines, and personal habits. It was also noted that with increasing age desynchrony becomes more likely, and the ability to deal with desynchronising events (such as jet lag) seems to decline. In old age desynchronised sleep–wake cycles can become self perpetuating, with disturbed night-time sleep resulting in extensive daytime napping which in turn affects night-time sleep. One obvious way in which the sleep–wake cycle can be strengthened, therefore, is through the maintenance of regular personal routines and habits. Regular times of going to bed and getting up, regular preparations for bedtime, and regularly scheduled daytime naps can all help to re-establish and maintain regular sleep–wake rhythms. As already described, incidentally, daytime naps assume a special significance in retirement and old age. While naps may be compensatory, making up for lost night-time sleep, they may also be a response to sheer boredom. If the latter, the nap itself represents a threat to the integrity of night-time sleep, and is therefore best avoided.

Regularity and sleep in dementia

Dementia has a particularly disruptive effect upon sleep, with prolonged daytime napping, frequent night-time awakenings and the added risk of confused nocturnal wandering. We have already noted, however, that sleeping drugs can actually increase the likelihood of confused behaviour especially in the frail and in those whose mental competence is already compromised. The maintenance of strict sleep–wake cycles, and the avoidance of excessive daytime sleeping seems particularly appropriate as an alternative or perhaps as an adjunct to drug therapy in the elderly mentally infirm.

The sleep environment

In the light of the research findings discussed in Chapter 3, three questions seem especially pertinent when assessing the sleep environment, which may not be a bedroom. First, is the sleep environment warm enough? Old and worn, though cherished bedding may be inefficient and need replacing. It might be advantageous to replace heavy combinations of sheets, blankets and counterpane, the weight of which can frequently aggravate painful joints, with lighter and more efficient duvets, quilts, or downies. Second, is the sleep environment quiet enough? As increasing age is associated with a progressive reduction in the auditory awakening threshold, the quietest possible environment is to be recommended. Previously preferred bedrooms in the front of the house overlooking the street, for example, might wisely be vacated for a quieter back bedroom. Finally, is the bed itself sufficiently comfortable? Older people are likely to sleep in older beds on older mattresses. Worn bedsprings and saggy mattresses can be detrimental to sound sleep, and can lead to joint aches and pains during the daytime. Excellent advice on what to look for in a new bed is provided by Professor Ian Oswald and Dr Kirstine Adam in their book *Get A Better Night's Sleep.*[12] Beds should provide even support for the entire body, and double beds should not 'dip' in the middle under the weight of two occupants.

Bedtime drinks

For many people, a drink at bedtime forms an intrinsic part of their pre-sleep behaviour, and many beverages have earned a reputation for promoting sleep. Nevertheless, as sleep changes with age it may become necessary to reconsider even well-established personal habits. If, for example, nocturia has become a problem, bedtime drinking is probably best avoided altogether. If, on the other hand, a bedtime drink is considered desirable it should be noted that caffeinated drinks (such as tea, coffee, cocoa, Pepsi Cola, Coca Cola, and Lucozade)[13] possess both stimulant and diuretic properties and may not be entirely suitable for those with fragile sleep. Malted milk drinks like 'Ovaltine' and 'Horlicks' have long been associated with 'good' sleep. While the research evidence suggests that this reputation is not entirely unfounded, it also suggests that the value of these drinks depends very much upon the dietary habits of the individual. In EEG laboratory studies conducted by Dr Kirstine Adam and Professor Ian Oswald, for example, it was found that among those accustomed to foods taken late at night, Horlicks was associated with better sleep (which, in this case, meant that sleep was longer and less broken). Conversely, among those unaccustomed to late night food, Horlicks at bedtime was associated with shorter, more broken sleep relative to that recorded on non-Horlicks nights.[14] Again, these findings reinforce the conclusion that the maintenance of consistent personal habits can optimise sleep quality (providing, of course, those personal habits are not in themselves detrimental to sleep).

Weight change and sleep

Before leaving the subject of food altogether, some comments on the relationship between weight and sleep are also relevant here. Some people emerge from middle age somewhat heavier than when they entered it and may, for cosmetic or health reasons, embark upon a programme of weight reduction. It has been shown by Professor Arthur Crisp and his colleagues at St George's Hospital Medical School in London that changes in weight can significantly affect quality of sleep. In studies of obese subjects losing weight, for example, significant weight loss was found to be associated with reduced total sleep and early morning awakening. Conversely, weight gain in those individuals with a history of anorexia nervosa (a condition characterised by self-imposed starvation) was associated with improved sleep and later awakening. In subsequent studies of different patient groups the point illustrated by these rather extreme examples has been confirmed – loss of weight can result in loss of sleep.[15]

Activity and exercise

While it might seem intuitively plausible that exercise facilitates sound sleep, research evidence for such a relationship is far from clear cut. In an extensive review of over 90 theoretical papers and experimental studies concerned with the effects of exercise upon sleep, Dr Jim Horne at the University of Loughborough concluded that non-athletes 'appear to show little, if any, sleep EEG effects following daytime exercise.'[16] Among highly-trained athletes, however, an increase in slow wave sleep has been observed on those nights which followed vigorous daily training sessions. During sleep EEG slow waves are associated with certain restorative processes, and it is likely that a change in this sleep stage is mediated by the body's need for restoration after the physiological wear and tear of training.

While the existence of elderly athletes must be acknowledged, the apparent benefits of such intense exercise (i.e. increases in slow waves) are of little practical relevance to most people in later life. There are, however, other ways in which exercise can influence sleep apart from its physiological cost. Many forms of moderate exercise can engender feelings which are themselves conducive to sleep, like tranquillity, personal satisfaction and wellbeing, and even sleepiness. As a source of both physical and intellectual stimulation, light exercise regularly taken can also help to offset the consequences of tedium which, as previously described, can be detrimental to sleep quality.

Evidence that general daytime stimulation can facilitate sleep is provided by an interesting study conducted at Dr Horne's laboratory at the University of Loughborough.[17] In a group of nine healthy young female students, sleep EEGs were recorded after two 'baseline' days of routine academic work in the library or laboratory, and after an 'experimental' day characterised by 'interest, variety and novelty', during which the student was taken to the zoo, an amusement park, and finally to the cinema in several cross-country car journeys. After the experimental day, volunteers were subjectively sleepier (as measured by a sleep questionnaire), fell asleep more rapidly, and showed longer periods of slow wave sleep than after the baseline days. Thus, whether perceived as exercise or not, activities which result in both mental and physical stimulation have implications for improved sleep quality (although it would be nice to see such experiments repeated using older volunteers). A word of caution is appropriate here. By definition, stimulating activities are incompatible with sleep and should, therefore, be discontinued well before bedtime (see the next section). Even in the young, exercise taken shortly before bedtime is more likely to disrupt sleep than facilitate it.

Pre-sleep mood

Ideally, two feelings should be obtained before retiring to bed: tiredness and personal calm. To go to bed without feeling tired is to invite a rather long sleep onset latency, while feelings of stress or anxiety can produce a state of mental and physical excitement incompatible with sleep. Methodical pre-sleep rituals (preparing for bed, preparing clothes for the morning, preparing for breakfast, etc.) can help here, and may actually serve as strategies for 'winding down' before finally getting into bed. Reading or perhaps listening to the radio in bed may also help to produce an optimal pre-sleep state of mind. As we shall see in the next section, however, under some circumstances, engaging in non sleep-related activities in bed (reading, for example) can actually be counter productive.

THE PSYCHOLOGICAL MANAGEMENT OF INSOMNIA

Over the past 20 years psychological research has contributed greatly to our understanding of the mechanisms which facilitate sleep. Based largely on findings derived from this research, clinical psychology has developed a variety of techniques and procedures which have proved extremely useful in the management of insomnia. Unlike hypnotic drugs, which are frequently prescribed without any real understanding of *why* the individual is experiencing poor sleep, these psychological treatments aim to identify and reduce the impact of factors which either cause or contribute to the insomnia. Two therapeutic approaches will be considered here. The first is based upon the concept of 'stimulus control', while the second utilises procedures which induce feelings of physical relaxation and mental calm. In both cases theory and therapy are inextricably linked, so in the sections which follow I will provide a brief account of both.

The treatment of insomnia through stimulus control

Many activities tend to occur in specific settings and under quite specific circumstances. (Sleep, for example, tends to occur in bed, in bedrooms, at night). Over time these settings and circumstances become signals, and sometimes quite powerful signals, for the behaviours associated with them. Once this relationship is well established, the presence of these signals (for example the bed, or the bedroom) actually makes the behaviour associated with them (i.e. sleep) much more likely. In psychological jargon a signal which sets the occasion for a particular behavioural response is called a 'discriminative stimulus', while the relationship which develops between the stimulus and the behavioural response it encourages is referred to as the 'stimulus control' of that behaviour. As already suggested sleep provides a good example of stimulus controlled behaviour, with the bed, the bedroom, or even perhaps the proximity of one's partner acting as signals for sleep onset.

The influence of environmental signals on sleep can, however, be weakened. For the insomniac lying awake in bed night after night, it is tempting to pass the time by reading, listening to the radio, smoking, etc. All of these activities are incompatible with sleep, and if repeated over time then bit by bit the stimuli which were once associated with rest and sleep become associated instead with wakefulness, and their ability to 'set the occasion' for sleeping diminishes. Thus, while loss of stimulus control may not be related to the onset of insomnia it may nevertheless contribute to the maintenance of insomnia. Stimulus control treatments, therefore, aim to re-establish the strength of those environmental events which serve as signals for sleep. In practice this means avoiding out of bed naps, going to bed only when sleepy, avoiding any activities unrelated to sleep in the bedroom (e.g. reading, listening to the radio, playing cards, etc.), and actually leaving the bedroom if the onset of sleep is delayed.

These techniques have been found to be extremely useful in the treatment of sleep onset insomnias although most of the published studies have concentrated on relatively young insomniacs.[18] Fortunately, elderly people have not been completely ignored. In 1983 a group of researchers at Washington University, St. Louis, reported that stimulus control procedures administered over a four week period substantially reduced the sleep onset latencies of 16 elderly volunteers whose ages ranged from 60 to 75 years.[19] Participants in this study were required to go to bed only when drowsy, to avoid any activity in the bedroom which was not associated with sleep (including worrying, eating, reading, etc.), and to leave the bed if awake for more than ten minutes (and not to return again unless drowsy). In addition, a sleep diary was maintained each day in which volunteers noted their frequency of awakening, difficulties in getting to, or returning to sleep, estimates of total sleep time, and their feelings of alertness in the morning. Of the 16 people who participated in the study, ten managed to reduce their sleep onset latency by 50 per cent or more. Furthermore, this improvement was still present when the volunteers were interviewed six weeks later. For some elderly people, then, stimulus control procedures can provide effective relief from lengthy and frustrating attempts to fall asleep.

The treatment of insomnia through relaxation

In 1967 Dr Lawrence J. Monroe of the University of Chicago published the results of a study in which selected psychological and physiological characteristics of self-described 'good' and 'poor' sleepers had been measured and compared. Both the good and the poor sleepers were recruited from the university community and, not surprisingly, comprised mainly young college students. Each of these volunteers spent two nights in the EEG sleep laboratory with sleep being recorded on the second night. (The first night was for adaptation; see Chapter 2.) When compared with the good sleepers, Dr Monroe found that the volunteers who described their usual sleep as poor actually slept less, were more restless during sleep, had higher body temperatures, and tended to have a faster pulse-rate. Overall, then, it looked as if poor sleepers were physiologically more active than good sleepers.[20] These results laid the foundations for the 'physiological-hyperactivity' theory of insomnia which suggested that insomniacs have more trouble than good sleepers in getting their bodies to relax. While subsequent studies have failed to find such clear-cut differences between good and poor sleepers, or have interpreted such findings in a different way (thus calling into question the validity of the theory),[18] clinical studies have shown that relaxation training can be of benefit in some types of insomnia.

Feelings of calm and tranquillity can be used to combat a variety of emotional problems, especially those associated with stress or anxiety. Over the years a number of self-help techniques have been developed which enable people to achieve states of sometimes quite profound relaxation. With the aid of a competent therapist, the individual is first trained in the use of a particular technique, and then encouraged to use it when circumstances demand. In much the same way as sleeping drugs are compared with placebos, the value of relaxation in the treatment of insomnia has been assessed by comparing real training programmes with 'dummy' treatments (i.e. some form of therapeutic contact not expected to affect sleep). Alternatively, some researchers have compared the sleep of those insomniacs who have received relaxation training with the sleep of insomniacs awaiting treatment (so-called 'waiting list' controls). In either case the results have shown that, where *getting* to sleep is the problem, relaxation methods can substantially reduce sleep onset latency and improve sleep quality.[18] Two of the most popularly used relaxation techniques, progressive muscle relaxation and autogenic training, are briefly outlined below. Not described here, but also effective in reducing sleep onset latency, are the many different forms of meditation, and the relaxation exercises associated with yoga.

Progressive muscle relaxation. Traditional methods of relaxing, such as simply flopping into a chair or onto a bed, are often unsatisfactory simply because we are not aware that our muscles are now 'relaxed'. Progressive muscle relaxation (or PMR) aims not only to relax tense muscles but also, and very importantly, aims to improve subjective awareness of this relaxation. Thus, subjects (who are lying in a comfortable position and in a suitably quiet environment) are required first to tense specific muscle groups, and then to release all tension, allowing the structures supported by those muscles to become limp and heavy. This tension-release cycle can last up to 50 seconds (5 seconds of tension followed by 45 seconds of release) for each muscle group, and is applied progressively to the muscle groups of the limbs, trunk, and even the face.

Autogenic training. While progressive muscle relaxation is targeted at the body, autogenic training is essentially a mental exercise during which the subject is encouraged to repeat, in a monotonous fashion, self-suggestions of physical heaviness alternating with suggestions of physical warmth. In a study reported by Perry Nicassio and Richard Bootzin of Northwestern University in the United States, for example, insomniacs were instructed to repeat the suggestion to themselves 'My right arm is heavy, I am at peace' several times before focusing attention on the other arm, the legs, etc. These self-suggestions of heaviness were then followed by similar self-suggestions of warmth 'My right arm is warm' etc.[21] In Nicassio and Bootzin's study, progressive muscle relaxation and autogenic training proved equally effective in reducing sleep onset latency and improving subjective sleep quality in a group of 30 insomniacs aged from 22 to 71 years. Both techniques are now well-established as treatments for sleep onset insomnia.

While the psychological techniques so far considered have been primarily concerned with sleep onset (i.e. *getting* to sleep), it will be remembered from Chapter 2 that one of the most frequently encountered problems among older insomniacs is sleep maintenance (i.e. *staying* asleep). A sleep maintenance problem can, of course, be considered as a problem in getting *back* to sleep, and as such may be influenced by some of the techniques already described. Nevertheless, this current focus upon sleep onset must be seen as one of the factors limiting the application of psychological treatments among elderly insomniacs. Where therapists have focused upon the characteristics of a whole night's sleep, it is clear, as we shall see in the next section, that some forms of psychological management can have a marked impact on sleep continuity.

Combined treatment programmes. Stimulus control and relaxation methods are derived from quite different theoretical backgrounds, and are assumed to work for quite different reasons. It is not unreasonable, therefore, to suggest that a combination of these two techniques might be more effective in the treatment of insomnia than either applied alone. In a small clinical study of three elderly volunteers with chronic insomnia, Ken Gledhill of St Luke's Hospital in Huddersfield, Yorkshire, assessed the value of a treatment 'package' comprising stimulus control and relaxation techniques in reducing sleep onset latency and intervening wakefulness.[22] After an initial period during which sleep diaries were completed, but no treatment was given, these volunteers were visited at home and provided with advice and instructions on stimulus control procedures similar to those described above. Unlike the St. Louis study, however, Gledhill did not ask his volunteers to leave their bedroom during periods of wakefulness at night. In addition, volunteers received training in autogenic relaxation, and were encouraged to practise the method once each day, and again at bedtime. This supervised instruction was continued each week over a 60 day period, during which time sleep diaries, in which the volunteers made a note of their estimated sleep onset latency, total sleep time, etc., were maintained daily.

The results from this study were presented not as averages but as trends for each of the three participants, thus providing a personal and very meaningful account of the impact of therapy.

Figure 6.1: Daily self-ratings of sleep onset latency from a 67 year old man practising autogenic relaxation and stimulus control techniques for poor sleep

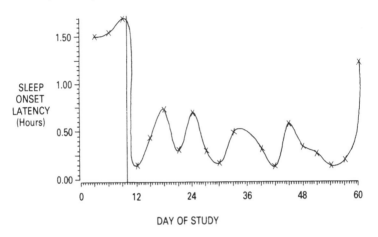

DAY OF STUDY

Note: Instruction began on day 8 (vertical line).
Source: Data from Gledhill, *Psychological Perspectives of Sleep and Sleep Problems in the Elderly Population; A Survey and Treatment Study*, Unpublished Master's Thesis, England, University of Leeds (1984).

Two of the three volunteers reported a decrease in sleep onset latency, a reduction in night-time awakenings, and an overall improvement in sleep quality during the study. Daily self-reports of sleep onset latency and sleep quality for one of these volunteers are shown in Figures 6.1 and 6.2 respectively. As much of this book has been concerned with averages and probabilities, this emphasis on the individual is, I think, particularly welcome. Before treatment, the man whose response to therapy is shown in Figures 6.1 and 6.2 was described as follows:

Mr H. was a 67 year old single man. Over a period of some years he found his sleep had worsened. Falling asleep frequently took an hour or longer while he would frequently wake 2 or 3 times in the night and have difficulty in getting back to sleep. Waking early in the morning was also a problem although it had been his normal practice when working to rise quite early. Mr H. felt that there was no obvious explanation for his sleep trouble. Apart from some

129

Figure 6.2: Daily self-ratings of sleep quality from a 67 year old man practising autogenic relaxation and stimulus control techniques for poor sleep

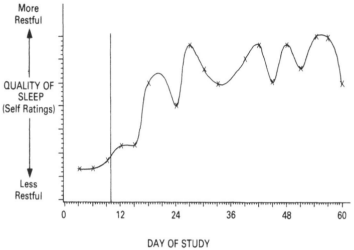

DAY OF STUDY

Note: Instruction began on day 8 (vertical line).
Source: Data from Gledhill, *Psychological Perspectives of Sleep and Sleep Problems in the Elderly Population; A Survey and Treatment Study*, Unpublished Master's Thesis, England, University of Leeds (1984).

mild hypertension [high blood pressure], he felt his health to be fine. His score on the Beck depression inventory [a questionnaire that assesses depression] was 6 [i.e. not depressed].

This person shows many of the 'normal' age-related changes in sleep described in Chapter 2. While both Figures show sometimes large fluctuations from day to day it is clear that Mr H. felt his sleep improve. [Apparently the sudden increase in sleep onset latency seen at about day 60 was only a temporary aberration, with sleep onset returning to its improved level shortly afterwards.] Of course, information concerning just one individual cannot be taken as a definitive evaluation of the therapy. Nevertheless, these preliminary results do indicate the possible value of therapeutic 'packages' in the treatment of insomnia in old age.

Cognitive therapies for poor sleep

For many years it was assumed that relaxation therapies were effective because insomniacs with sleep onset problems were in some way physiologically overactive, and therefore benefited from help in 'slowing down' at the end of the day. Since the publication of Monroe's results in 1967, however, several studies have failed to find any consistent physiological differences between good and poor sleepers, suggesting that hyperactivity theory is an inadequate explanation of sleep-onset insomnia. If this is the case, why should relaxation therapies with their emphasis on physical calmness work at all? In recent years psychologists have increasingly turned their attention to pre-sleep thoughts as a possible cause of sleep onset problems, and many have come to the conclusion that often it is mental not physical overactivity which keeps people awake.

Some insomniacs appear to have a problem controlling their pre-sleep thoughts and find it difficult to create the optimal pre-sleep state of mind described above. For these people relaxation therapy might work not because it slows down the body but because, by providing a focus of attention, it prevents the uncontrollable and intrusive thoughts which can delay sleep onset. The cognitive origins of insomnia (psychologists describe bodily processes as 'behavioural' and mental processes as 'cognitive') have yet to be adequately researched, but it seems likely that individuals can be taught a variety of methods for dealing with thoughts incompatible with sleep.

In a small exploratory study conducted at St George's Hospital Medical School in London, Maureen Tomeny, a clinical psychologist, taught a group of ten chronic sleep onset insomniacs (the oldest of whom was 62) a number of strategies for recognising and challenging the type of pre-sleep ruminations which maintain wakefulness. The volunteers were encouraged to judge whether their thoughts concerning guilt, fear, low self-esteem, or even thoughts concerned with what they had to do the next day were exaggerated, unrealistic, or irrational.[23] In this way, they learned to exercise control over their intrusive thoughts, and to replace them with reassuring and rational alternatives. Over five weeks of therapy these volunteers reported reductions in both sleep onset latency, and the frequency of night-time awakenings. Among elderly people who, because of infirmity (arthritis or stroke victims, for example) find the emphasis on muscle tension and relaxation problematical, such cognitive therapies for poor sleep, when fully developed, may offer an effective alternative.

ALTERNATIVES TO HYPNOTIC DRUGS IN HOSPITALS

Where the hospital environment is the probable cause of sleep disturbance, it is, of course, logical to attend first to the noise, temperature, light intensity, etc., before prescribing for the patient. Where sleep problems persist, hypnotics can still be avoided. In a study reported by Dr A.J. Bayer and Professor M.S.J. Pathy of the Department of Geriatric Medicine, University of Wales, requests from elderly patients for hypnotic drugs were treated in the following way. Wherever possible, the patient's existing sedative drugs, or drugs with sedative properties (for example, antidepressants) were re-scheduled in order to maximise the sedative effect at night. Where a physical cause of poor sleep was evident, for example pain or breathlessness, this was appropriately treated without hypnotics.

Complaining patients were also offered advice and reassurance by the medical and nursing staff. Then, if the sleep problem continued, patients were given an inactive placebo tablet which, they were told, was a hypnotic called 'Danos' (a name derived from the Welsh for 'night'). If this 'drug' proved unsatisfactory, it was replaced by a genuine hypnotic. The study was conducted in two wards where, over a 12 month period, 390 patients requested sleeping pills. Of these 37 (9.5 per cent) were satisfied without the prescription of additional drugs, while 216 (55.4 per cent) patients were 'entirely satisfied' with placebo capsules. Only 137 (35.1 per cent) of these patients eventually received an active hypnotic.[24] On a larger scale, the use of dummy drugs and clinical deception may be both practically and ethically unacceptable. Nevertheless, this study clearly demonstrates the value of an imaginative and flexible response to complaints of poor sleep in hospital.

SUMMARY

It is now widely acknowledged that hypnotics are unsuitable for the continuous long term treatment of insomnia, especially in older people. While alternative therapeutic approaches require a more thoughtful and flexible response to complaints of poor sleep in later life, the clinical and research evidence indicates that such alternatives are both practical and effective. Many of the factors which contribute to insomnia in later life are themselves amenable to treatment, and provide a target for rational alternatives to the use of hypnotic drugs. For example, where disturbed sleep is secondary to a medical or psychiatric disorder, specific treatment for the underlying cause is often more appropriate than the symptomatic treatment of insomnia. Whether or not a specific underlying cause is identified, habits and behaviours known to be detrimental to sleep should be avoided. In particular, the maintenance of regular personal routines such as bedtime, mealtimes, exercise, etc. can help to minimise the impact of age on the sleep–wake cycle. Psychological treatments have also proved useful in the treatment of insomnia, particularly sleep onset insomnias (i.e. trouble *getting* to sleep), and may provide a positive alternative to the use of hypnotics. While stimulus control and relaxation techniques have been shown to improve subjective sleep quality in younger insomniacs, what little evidence there is suggests that these techniques can also be successfully employed in the treatment of elderly people.

NOTES AND REFERENCES

1. Committee on the Review of Medicines, 'Systematic Review of the Benzodiazepines', *British Medical Journal*, 1 (1980) pp. 910–12
2. W. Dement, W. Seidel and M. Carskadon, 'Daytime Alertness, Insomnia and Benzodiazepines', *Sleep*, 5 (1982) pp. 528–45
3. This type of insomnia is explicitly recognised in the Association of Sleep Disorders Center's 'Outline and Diagnostic Classification of Sleep and Arousal Disorders', *Sleep*, 2(1) (1979)
4. H.S. Jones and I. Oswald, 'Two Cases of Healthy Insomnia', *Electroencephalography and Clinical Neurophysiology*, 24 (1968) pp. 378–80
5. I. Oswald, 'Sleep Disorders', in R.E. Kendell and A.K. Zealley (eds), *Companion to Psychiatric Studies*, Edinburgh, Churchill Livingstone (1983)
6. A. Kales and J.D. Kales, *Evaluation and Treatment of Insomnia*, New York, Oxford University Press (1984)
7. 'Hypnotics and Hangover', *British Medical Journal*, 1 (1980) p. 743
8. D.F. Kripke, S. Ancoli-Israel and N. Okudaira, 'Sleep Apnea

and Nocturnal Myoclonus in the Elderly', *Neurobiology of Aging*, 3 (1982) pp. 329–36

9. K. Jones and C.M. Castleden, 'A Double-Blind Comparison of Quinine Sulphate and Placebo in Muscle Cramps', *Age and Ageing*, 12 (1983) pp. 155–8

10. G.V. Stimson, 'Doctor-Patient Interaction and some Problems for Prescribing', *Journal of the Royal College of General Practitioners*, 26, supplement 1 (1976) pp. 88–96

11. N. Kleitman, *Sleep and Wakefulness*, Chicago, University of Chicago Press (1963)

12. I. Oswald and K. Adam, *Get a Better Night's Sleep*, London, Martin Dunitz (1983)

13. For an assessment of caffeine levels in Pepsi Cola, Coca Cola, and Lucozade, see A. Darragh, R.F. Lambe, D. Hallinhan and D.A. O'Kelly, 'Caffeine in Soft Drinks', *Lancet*, 1 (1979) p. 1196

14. K. Adam, 'Dietary Habits and Sleep after Bedtime Food Drinks', *Sleep*, 3(1) (1980) pp. 47–58

15. For a review of this research see A. Crisp, 'Sleep, Activity, Nutrition and Mood', *British Journal of Psychiatry*, 137 (1980) pp. 1–7

16. J.A. Horne, 'The Effects of Exercise upon Sleep: A Critical Review', *Biological Psychology*, 12 (1981) pp. 241–90

17. J.A. Horne and A. Minard, 'Sleep and Sleepiness Following a Behaviourally "Active" Day', Ergonomics, 28(3) (1985) pp. 567–75

18. For an excellent discussion of theoretical issues in, and psychological treatments of insomnia see T.D. Borkovec, 'Insomnia', *Journal of Consulting and Clinical Psychology*, 50, 6 (1982) pp. 880–95

19. R. Puder, P. Lacks, A.D. Bertelson and M. Storandt, 'Short-Term Stimulus Control Treatment of Insomnia in Older Adults', *Behaviour Therapy*, 14 (1983) pp. 424–9

20. L.J. Monroe, 'Psychological and Physiological Differences between Good and Poor Sleepers', *Journal of Abnormal Psychology*, 72(3) (1967) pp. 255–64

21. P. Nicassio and R. Bootzin, 'A Comparison of Progressive Relaxation and Autogenic Training as Treatments for Insomnia', *Journal of Abnormal Psychology*, 83(3) (1974) pp. 253–60

22. K. Gledhill, 'Psychological Perspectives of Sleep and Sleep Problems in the Elderly Population; A Survey and Treatment Study', Unpublished Master's Thesis, University of Leeds, England (1984)

23. M. Tomeny, 'A Comparison of Relaxation and Cognitive Therapy for Insomnia', Unpublished Master's Thesis, University of Surrey, England (1984)

24. A.J. Bayer and M.S.J. Pathy, 'Requests for Hypnotic Drugs and Placebo Response in Elderly Hospital In-patients', *Postgraduate Medical Journal*, 61 (1985) pp. 317–20

7

Notes on Dreaming

Since Aserinsky and Kleitman's discovery of REM sleep in 1953[1] (see Chapter 1), and subsequent demonstrations that it was during the REM stage that most dreaming occurs, dream research, as distinct from sleep research, has become an increasingly specialised field of study. While interest in sleeping and dreaming can be considered to 'overlap' in the area of REM sleep, studies of dreaming with their emphasis on the content, function, and interpretation of dream experiences, extend well beyond the EEG laboratory, and well beyond the intended scope of this book. Nevertheless, without going too far out of the depth set in earlier chapters it is possible to comment, using terms of reference already defined, on two aspects of dreaming in old age, namely the recall of dreams, and the content of dreams. While this discussion will be limited to only a handful of studies it is interesting to note that, like sleep research before it, dream research has tended to focus upon children and young adults to the exclusion of the middle aged and the elderly, and even now there is a dearth of information on dreaming in later life. (Freud, for example, had virtually nothing to say on the subject of dreams in old age.)

DREAM RECALL IN OLD AGE

The relationship between REM sleep and the occurrence of dreams has been established through a fairly straightforward experimental procedure. Connect volunteers to an EEG machine, wait for them to fall asleep, then awaken them during a defined sleep stage and ask them if they were dreaming. In this way it has been found that while over 80 per cent of REM awakenings in young adults are associated with dream recall, NREM awakenings are associated with much lower levels of dream recall and, in some studies, with no dream recall at all.[2] As is clearly shown in Figure 2.6, however, total amounts of REM sleep decrease steadily throughout life. The consequences of this age-related decline are also clear; elderly people not only spend less time sleeping than young people, they also spend less time dreaming.

In addition to this absolute reduction in the amount of 'dreaming' sleep, EEG laboratory studies also indicate that in elderly volunteers dreams are less likely to be remembered following REM awakenings. Assessing dream recall in both young and elderly volunteers, Drs Edwin Kahn and Charles Fisher found that while 87 per cent of REM awakenings were associated with the recall of coherent dreams in young volunteers,[3] dreams of a similar quality were reported in only 45.2 per cent of such awakenings in a group of 27 volunteers aged 66 – 87.[4] (Elderly women, it was found, were more likely than elderly men to recall their dreams.) These laboratory findings seem to be in agreement with day-to-day experiences of dreaming. Thus, in a survey of sleep and dreaming conducted among 260 women aged 30 – 79, and 460 men aged 21 – 81 Dr Harold Zepelin found that dreams were least frequently recalled among those aged 50 years and over.[5] Why, then, should dream recall decline with age? Perhaps, subconsciously, older people are better at repressing their dream experiences,[6] or perhaps the older and wiser are simply less eager than the young to externalise their stream of consciousness. Of course, it is also possible that as a general consequence of declining memory, dreams just become more difficult to remember. Whatever the reason, it does seem to be the case that for many people, dream experiences become less common with increasing age.

DREAM CONTENT IN OLD AGE

Studies of the dream content in elderly people have mostly been conducted within the framework of psychoanalytical theory which, after the teachings of Freud, draws a distinction between the 'manifest' content of the dream (i.e. what we actually remember dreaming) and the 'latent' content of the dream (i.e. what we are *really* dreaming about). Through a process which Freud termed 'dream work', potentially disturbing conflicts and memories which arise in the unconscious mind and which form the latent content of our dreams are converted into mostly harmless though bizarre dream sequences — the manifest content. In this way dreams act as the 'guardians of sleep', masking the hidden conflicts which would otherwise awaken us. Dream work is not haphazard but appears rather to be an organised, even lawful process during which certain thoughts, conflicts, and fears are given symbolic rather than literal expression.

In two separate studies reported in 1961 and 1963, Drs Altshuler, Barad, and Goldfarb of New York found that the manifest content of dreams in both institutionalised[7] and non-institutionalised[8] elderly people (as reported during weekly interviews) was characterised by the themes of helplessness, vulnerability, and diminished physical and material resources. According to Dr Altshuler and his colleagues these themes were evident in dreams concerning hunger, being threatened or attacked, or of being lost in a strange place, all of which were repeatedly described by the elderly people taking part in this study. It was also found that dreams with a high sexual content were not infrequent, though according to these authors, the relevance of the sexual symbolism was different for males and females. In elderly men, sexual dreams tended to reiterate the theme of anxiety, failure, and diminished performance. Among elderly women, on the other hand, dreams with a high sexual content tended to be associated with pleasurable gratification and personal security; one woman, for example, reported a 'sexy dream' in which she was 'kept' by a rich young man, apparently reflecting the themes of need for and provision of help.[8]

The rather gloomy conclusions of Drs Altshuler, Barad and Goldfarb, (i.e. that the dreams of elderly people are characterised by such themes as loss, weakness and vulnerability) are not entirely supported by other researchers. In the REM awakening study mentioned above, Drs Kahn and Fisher found no evidence that the dreams of their elderly volunteers were preoccupied with frustration or loss. An important factor which may have contributed to these different findings concerns the way in which the dreams were recorded. Unlike the REM awakenings of Kahn and Fisher, Dr Altshuler and his colleagues relied on daytime recall covering all the dreams of the previous week. It has been suggested that over such a period of time night dreams and day dreams become confused, and what is actually recalled is not a 'pure' REM dream, but rather an accumulation of conscious and dream experiences.[3] It might also be the case that, over several weekly interviews, interviewers can actually influence the very dreams they are asking their interviewees to recall. Put another way, if you expect reports of dreams preoccupied with loss and vulnerability, then, by communicating this expectation to the dreamer, you may well get reports of dreams preoccupied with loss and vulnerability. Dr Altshuler and his colleagues did find that after several consecutive interviews the elderly participants in their study began to report dreams which had included the interviewing psychiatrist.

Finally, something of the complexity of dream content analysis in relation to age can be gained from a study reported in 1964 by Dr M.E. Smith and Dr C. Hall, in which the life-long dream diaries of an elderly woman (at that time aged 77) were examined.[9] The owner of the diaries, herself a psychologist, had recorded her dreams since the age of 25 and, over the years, had accumulated some 649 detailed dream descriptions. No less than 52 of these dreams were recorded in her 75th year! (Illustrating the point made in earlier chapters that while 'on average' certain events — diminishing dream recall, for instance — become more likely with increasing age, there are always exceptions.) A particularly interesting finding from Smith and Hall's analysis is that, while the themes of vulnerability and loss (as described by Dr Altshuler and his colleagues) are indeed present among the 649 dream reports, it appeared that these were as likely to occur in the earlier (younger) dreams as in the later. They conclude that 'At every age, dreams reveal considerable inadequacy and helplessness on the part of the dreamer'. Thus, Drs Smith and Hall found that the theme of eating (associated with weakness by Dr Altshuler and his colleagues) was indeed frequently reported by their subject in old age, occurring in 25 per cent of this woman's dreams after the age of 70. However, the same theme occurred almost as frequently in dreams reported before the age of 46.

Dream content and its interpretation is a complex and contentious subject, and it would be unwise even to attempt a conclusion on the basis of the few studies described here. It is not unreasonable, however, to suggest that while some people (the subject of Smith and Hall's study, for instance), regard dreaming as an important and essential part of their mental life, others regard dreaming as an occasionally interesting mental side-show, the importance of which should not be over-rated. Perhaps, then, as we age, the content and recall of our dreams are positively influenced by the importance we have attached to them. It would be nice to think that such a process would lead ultimately to an equitable distribution of dream experiences in old age, with those who value dreams recalling them, and those who place a lower value on dreams recalling them less often. This, of course, is just the sort of theory which research can resolve.

NOTES AND REFERENCES

1. E. Aserinsky and N. Kleitman, 'Regularly Occurring Periods of Eye Movement and Concomitant Phenomena During Sleep', *Science*, 118 (1953) pp. 273–4
2. See R.J. Berger, 'The Sleep and Dream Cycle', reprinted in S.G.M. Lee and A.R. Mayes (eds), *Dreams and Dreaming: Selected Readings*, Harmondsworth, Penguin (1973)
3. E. Kahn, C. Fisher and L. Lieberman, 'Dream Recall in the Normal Aged', *Journal of the American Geriatrics Society*, 17 (1969) pp. 1121–6
4. E. Kahn, W. Dement, C. Fisher and J.E. Barmack, 'Incidence of Color in Immediately Recalled Dreams', *Science*, 137 (1962) pp. 1054–5
5. H. Zepelin, 'A Survey of Age Differences in Sleep Patterns and Dream Recall among Well-Educated Men and Women', *Sleep Research*, 2 (1973) p. 81
6. The term 'repression' is Freudian and refers to that process whereby emotionally discomforting thoughts are 'pushed' out of consciousness and into unconsciousness.
7. M. Barad, K.Z. Altshuler and A.I. Goldfarb, 'A Survey of Dreams in Aged Persons', *Archives of General Psychiatry*, 4 (1961) pp. 419–24
8. K.Z. Altshuler, M. Barad and A.I. Goldfarb, 'A Survey of Dreams in the Aged. Part II: Noninstitutionalized Subjects', *Archives of General Psychiatry*, 8 (1963) pp. 33–7
9. M.E. Smith and C. Hall, 'An Investigation of Regression in a Long Dream Series', *Journal of Gerontology*, 19 (1964) pp. 66–71

8

Responding to Insomnia
in Later Life

The organisation of this book clearly reflects the degree to which issues relevant to sleep and ageing are divided between changes in the structure and quality of sleep on one hand, and the social response to these changes on the other. In fact, the response occurs at two different levels. First there is the personal response where we judge such changes to be expected, unexpected, tolerable or intolerable, etc. before presumably acting in accordance with these judgements. If changes in our sleep are judged by us to be unexpected, intolerable or just generally unwelcome, we may seek advice or help from those whom society considers qualified to give it. At this point we engage the second level of response, that from professional carers, which generally means a medical practitioner. Much of the information considered in the latter part of this book allows the conclusion that at both levels, a characteristic style of responding has evolved. At the personal level, vast numbers of people apparently judge the age-related changes in their sleep to be at best unexpected and at worst unacceptable, as evidenced by the number of older adults who express dissatisfaction with their sleep during medical consultations. At the professional level, it is also clear that a medical tradition has developed which seems to assume that insomnia[1] in old age is often due to some form of benzodiazepine deficiency. In this final chapter I would like to discuss some of the factors which currently support these styles of responding, and then consider the likelihood of change both in the personal and in the professional response to sleep and ageing.

THE PERSONAL RESPONSE

Alterations in sleep represent just a single (and not necessarily the most important) component in the complex sequence of biological, psychological, and social changes which collectively make up the ageing process. How we respond to these changes is greatly influenced by our understanding of them and by our expectations of ageing in general. For example, most adults do not regard the appearance of grey hair as a sign of illness requiring medical attention. Rather, greying hair is an age-related event for which we are socially (though perhaps not emotionally) prepared. Specifically, we recognise the event as 'normal', while in general we also recognise the context (ageing) in which it occurs. However, relative to some aspects of ageing (like greying hair, or reductions in physical speed, or changes in skin texture) alterations in sleep quality are socially inconspicuous. For this reason expectations of sleep are more likely to be influenced by inherited or 'common' knowledge rather than by direct observation. It is interesting to note, therefore, that much conventional wisdom about sleep, as contained in popular maxims, seems to assume a quite unrealistic (and misleading) life-long stability in sleeping patterns. For example, such pearls as 'early to bed, early to rise . . .' etc., or 'an hour before midnight is worth more than one hour after midnight'[2] are of little value to elderly people who would be better advised to go to bed as late as possible so that their sleep stretches at least till dawn. (And does a satisfying daytime nap count as before or after midnight?)

In much the same way the commonly held belief that around eight hours sleep per night is a universal norm for adult human beings also does little to prepare anyone for the declining total sleep time so characteristic of growing old. This particular item of mis-information can pop up in the most incongruous places. For example, in an otherwise helpful book intended for those 'Caring for an elderly relative', Dr Keith Thompson asserts that 'Most people need about seven or eight hours' sleep at night'.[3] Most young people might, most elderly people certainly *do not*. Again, in addition to its factual inaccuracy the statement reinforces the assumption that, in adult life, sleeping patterns remain stable. It would, of course, be over simplistic to suggest that unrealistic expectations (from whatever cause) represent the only factor influencing the personal response to sleep and ageing. It is nevertheless reasonable to suppose that an unexpected and misunderstood event is more likely to be interpreted as abnormal, a view which is often reinforced by the medical response to complaints of poor sleep in later life.

The socially acquired notion of doing 'the right thing' also influences the personal response. Here the medicalisation of society, the welfare state (in Britain), the behaviour of our role models which we observe and emulate, and other factors encourage us to take our complaint to a medical practitioner for assessment. Not to do so might actually result in a sense of irresponsibility.

THE MEDICAL RESPONSE

It is remarkable that while events which influence sleep diversity with increasing age (see Chapters 2 and 3), the medical response to disturbed sleep is fairly uniform for all age groups. Thus, the prescription of hypnotic drugs is the principal, and often the only, medical response to insomnia whether the patient is young, middle-aged, or elderly. Undoubtedly one of the main factors contributing to this pharmacological preference is the existence of safe and effective benzodiazepine hypnotics, the prescribing of which is quick, simple, often cheap, and very importantly quintessentially medical. However, the problems associated with these drugs (see Chapter 5) are not about to go away, and the need for a broader, more flexible response is increasingly being recognised, not least by the consumers themselves. Non-pharmacological alternatives, on the other hand, are slow, complex, consume more resources and, another very important point, are not exclusively 'medical'. It is not too difficult to see, therefore, that a therapeutically flexible approach to the management of insomnia in later life might require a shift in prevailing medical attitudes.

It would be inaccurate to suggest that medicine shows a consistent hostility towards alternative non-pharmacological approaches to the treatment of insomnia in old age. Nevertheless, a 'medical attitude' which reflects a preference amounting almost to a prejudice in favour of pharmacological treatments not infrequently appears in the medical literature. In a recently published comprehensive textbook of geriatric medicine, for example, Drs Spiegel and Azcona devote almost one-fifth of their chapter on 'Sleep and its disorders' to a description of drug therapy for sleeplessness. These authors then offer a very much shorter account of non-pharmacological therapies (including relaxation and behaviour therapies) for insomnia which is introduced with the following statement:

> There are numerous recommended ways of inducing sleep without resorting to drugs, although many of these supposedly effective methods contradict one another.[4]

In political circles, such an approach could be construed as trashing the opposition without presenting an argument!

In many ways, the combination of the personal and the professional response (often in the consulting room or surgery) reflects in microcosm the relationship between society and the medical enterprise it supports. This relationship is built upon numerous assumptions from both participants. The doctor makes assumptions about what the patient wants and the patient makes assumptions about what the doctor can reasonably do. Both, however, influence each other's assumptions. Thus, many doctors are convinced that their insomniac patients only want sleeping tablets, while many patients hold their hypnotics to be proof positive that they are suffering from a medical disorder. As regards the prescription of hypnotic drugs, then, I think it would be quite wrong to suggest that the medical profession imposes its professional response upon its patients. Rather, in collaborating with and contributing to that response, it could be argued that the consumers get the medicine they deserve. However, many of the assumptions underlying both the personal and professional responses are changing, and in the next section I would like finally to consider the impact this may have on the overall social response to sleep and ageing.

SCOPE FOR CHANGE

Attitudes towards illness and medicine are not unrelated to age. It has often been pointed out, for example, that the circumstances in which the present elderly generation grew up have produced a stoicism in the older members of society not seen in the young. It is also the case that medicine has achieved its present social and scientific stature during the lifetime of today's elderly generation who, perhaps as a result, have high expectations of medicine, and no small amount of trust in medical practitioners. This latter image of medicine, and the attitude which seems to accompany it is, I think, changing fairly rapidly. Recent years have seen a slowing down in medical achievements at least in so far as they affect most members of the general public. In addition, a whole generation has now grown up which, primed by the thalidomide disaster of the early 1960s, has come to realise that technological medicine brings high risks and sometimes dubious benefits. It is likely, therefore, that the unquestioning faith of earlier generations is being replaced by a cautious and inquisitive respect for medical technology. Perhaps as a consequence of this process of social education sleeping tablets will not in future be received so enthusiastically without a full description of their effects, side-effects and pedigree.

In addition to changes in the perceived status of medicine, current social attitudes towards health which place a greater emphasis on self-help and personal maintenance, are preparing future elderly generations for a more self-reliant old age. This shift in attitude is particularly well illustrated by the interest currently being shown in alternative or complementary therapies, many of which emphasise the active participation of the individual in the process of healing. (One of the major benefits of the psychological therapies discussed in Chapter 6 is the rewarding feeling of personal *control* over sleep achieved by some insomniacs.) Clearly, many people want to take a more active part in maintaining their health and, as such attitudes become more prevalent, will be less likely to be contented with the offer of a pill for every ill, preferring instead an explanation. It is also likely that future elderly generations will have an overall better understanding, and clearer expectations of old age. In this they may well be assisted not only by education and a growing popular literature on middle and late life, but also by the direct experience of growing up in an ageing society, an advantage not enjoyed by those currently in their seventies and older.

These changes in attitude among the consumers of health care find an echo within the medical profession itself. The development of holistic medicine (which emphasises the uniqueness and physical integrity of the individual instead of reducing patients to the level of a diseased organ or a malfunctioning system) and a growing interest in alternative or complementary therapeutic systems (for example, acupuncture, homeopathy, and osteopathy) are indicative of this new medical mood. Also indicative of a new mood within medicine is a growing willingness to re-analyse issues relating to hypnotic drug use not only in terms of which hypnotic to prescribe, but also in terms of a more fundamental clinical decision, whether to prescribe something or whether to prescribe nothing. In an article published in the *British Medical Journal* in 1985, for example, Dr A.C. Higgit and colleagues suggested that benzodiazepine drugs should not be prescribed when the cause of the complaint appears to be a transient emotional trauma (e.g. bereavement, divorce) because of the risk of dependence.

In brief, the argument presented here may be summarised as follows. Ideally, the therapeutic approach to complaints of poor sleep in old age should be broadly based (comprising many treatment approaches including the judicious use of hypnotic drugs) and flexible, able to adjust to the needs of the patient. While the personal response to sleep and ageing operates to place the individual in contact with medical practitioners, the medical response is all too often narrow and inflexible. This state of affairs is supported by the attitudes of the patient, the prevailing attitudes within medicine, and the relationship which currently exists between elderly consumers of care and the medical profession itself. Neither the attitudes nor the relationship are immutable. Forces operating within society at large are currently changing the way patients regard medicine and therapeutic drug use. Forces operating within medicine are currently changing the way doctors regard non-pharmacological treatment approaches. As the younger patients age, the 'new' elderly generation will enter late life with different expectations and will require a different style of care.

Changes in attitudes towards medicine, and changes in medical attitudes towards patients will not, of course, change the biological events which so often mediate complaints of poor sleep in old age. Neither will these changes affect the pathological sleep disorders which will continue to require specialist medical intervention. Alterations in attitude can, however, alter the way such events are perceived, interpreted, and dealt with. Imagine a theoretical threshold above which an event merits (according to our own criteria) medical attention, and below which an event is recognised as an aspect of life with which we can deal ourselves; the overall effect of these changes will be to raise this threshold with regard to sleep. How far and how quickly will be determined by the magnitude and speed of social change.

NOTES AND REFERENCES

1. As in Chapter 6 'insomnia' is regarded here as the complaint of poor sleep

2. This particular maxim has regional variants, with the exchange-rate for a pre-midnight hour sometimes as high as two post-midnight hours

3. M.K. Thompson, *Caring for an Elderly Relative; A Guide To Home Care*, London, Martin Dunitz (1986)

4. R. Spiegel and A. Azcona, 'Sleep and its Disorders', in M.S.J. Pathy (ed.), *Principles and Practice of Geriatric Medicine*, John Wiley and Sons Ltd, Chichester and New York (1985)

5. A.C. Higgit, M.H. Lader and P. Fonagy, 'Clinical Management of Benzodiazepine Dependence', *British Medical Journal*, 291 (1985) pp. 688–90

Name Index

Subject Index

hospitals, and noise 70–1
  and hypnotic drug use 85–6,
    89–90, 132
hypertension 59
hypnogram 11
hypnotic drugs, daytime
    withdrawal 108–10
  effects of 77–84
  residual and cumulative
    effects 100–5
  withdrawal 59, 106–8
hypnotic drug use, 84–95
  see also hospitals, residential
    homes, sex differences

iatrogenic causes of
    sleeplessness 57–60
insomnia 117
  medical response to 142–3
  personal response to 141–2
  physiological-hyperactivity
    theory of 126
  see also quality of sleep
institutionalisation 69–71
intervening wakefulness 10
  age-related changes 28–9
  and hypnotic drugs 80

jet lag 15
  see also transmeridian travel

loneliness 66–8
loprazolam 80, 81, 83, 103,
    106–7, 109
lorazepam 83
lormetazepam 83, 103–4

midazolam 110
mood and sleep 67, 123–4
multiple sleep latency test
    (MSLT) 15
  see also sleepiness

napping, age-related trends in
    34–7
  daytime sleepiness 38–40
  instrumentally recorded 36
  total 24 hour sleep 40–1
nightmares, and drug use 59
  and REM rebound 107–8

nitrazepam 78, 79, 83, 101–4,
    105
nocturia 49–51
nocturnal cramp 56
  treatment 118
nocturnal myoclonus see
    periodic movements in sleep
noise 33–4, 120–1
  see also hospitals
NREM sleep 8
  age-related changes 30

obesity, sleep apnoea 51–2, 55
  snoring 55
  see also weight change and
    sleep
oxazepam 83

pain and discomfort 56–7
paradoxical sleep see rapid eye
    movement sleep
penile erections, in REM sleep
    8–9
  night-time awakenings and
    29
periodic movements in sleep
    (PMS) 55–6
  treatment 118
placebo 80
polysomnogram 7–9
poverty 68–9
  see also bedroom
    temperature
progressive muscle relaxation
  see relaxation therapy
psychological therapies for
    insomnia 124–32
psychotropic drugs 84

quality of sleep, age-related
    changes in 22–5
  measurement of 12–14
  hypnotic drugs and 80–2
questionnaire surveys of sleep
    22–5
quinine sulphate 118

rapid eye movement (REM)
    sleep, 6–7, 8, 30
  and dreams 6–7, 135–6